INTERNAL FAMILY SYSTEMS THERAPY
FOR SHAME AND GUILT

Also from Martha Sweezy

Internal Family Systems Therapy,
Second Edition
Richard C. Schwartz and Martha Sweezy

Internal Family Systems Therapy for Shame and Guilt

Martha Sweezy

Foreword by Richard C. Schwartz

THE GUILFORD PRESS
New York   London

The author has checked with sources believed to be reliable in her efforts to provide
information that is complete and generally in accord with the standards of practice
that are accepted at the time of publication. However, in view of the possibility of
human error or changes in behavioral, mental health, or medical sciences, neither the
author, nor the editors and publisher, nor any other party who has been involved in
the preparation or publication of this work warrants that the information contained
herein is in every respect accurate or complete, and they are not responsible for any
errors or omissions or the results obtained from the use of such information. Readers
are encouraged to confirm the information contained in this book with other sources.

Library of Congress Cataloging-in-Publication Data

Names: Sweezy, Martha, author.
Title: Internal family systems therapy for shame and guilt / Martha Sweezy.
Description: New York : The Guilford Press, [2023] | Includes
    bibliographical references and index.
Identifiers: LCCN 2022057886 | ISBN 9781462552467 (paperback) |
    ISBN 9781462552474 (cloth)
Subjects: LCSH: Shame. | Family psychotherapy.
Classification: LCC BF575.S45 S85 2023 | DDC 152.4/4—dc23/eng/20230415
LC record available at *https://lccn.loc.gov/2022057886*

I dedicate this book to the next generation of psychotherapists,
including my daughter, Theo Sweezy,
and our dear young Swedish friend and colleague, Kristin Palme.
I trust you will start where my generation leaves off
and make your own great discoveries.
I hope this book helps.

About the Author

Martha Sweezy, PhD, is Assistant Professor in Psychiatry at Harvard Medical School, part-time, and Research, Training, and Curriculum Consultant at the Center for Mindfulness and Compassion, Cambridge Health Alliance, where she consults and is supervising in a study using Internal Family Systems (IFS) groups to treat posttraumatic stress disorder. She teaches on IFS, shame, and guilt nationally and internationally, and has a private psychotherapy practice. Dr. Sweezy has published articles in peer-reviewed journals and has coedited or coauthored several books and treatment manuals on IFS.

About the Author

Martha Sweezy, PhD, is Assistant Professor of Psychiatry at Harvard Medical School, part-time, and Research, Training, and Curriculum Consultant at the Center for Mindfulness and Compassion, Cambridge Health Alliance, where she consults and is supervising in a study using Internal Family Systems (IFS) groups to treat posttraumatic stress disorder. She teaches on IFS, shame, and guilt nationally and internationally, and has a private psychotherapy practice. Dr. Sweezy has published articles in peer-reviewed journals and has coedited or coauthored several books and treatment manuals on IFS.

Foreword

Even before writing this book, Martha Sweezy had made great contributions to Internal Family Systems (IFS; the therapy approach I developed that embraces psychic multiplicity as the norm) with her writing, editing, and teaching. Martha and I met in Cambridge, Massachusetts, in 2005, when she attended one of my lectures on IFS. She received training in IFS right away, and we began collaborating (with Nancy Sowell and Larry Rosenberg) to teach IFS to staff and trainees in the Department of Psychiatry of the Cambridge Health Alliance (CHA), which serves an economically, ethnically, racially, and diagnostically diverse population and has long been a national model for community mental health. We also started writing together. Most recently, we coauthored the foundational text *Internal Family Systems Therapy, Second Edition*. We continue to write together and teach IFS at CHA, which I am proud to say has adopted IFS as one of its primary treatment modalities and which, with Zev Schuman-Olivier's leadership, is conducting important research on IFS as a treatment for posttraumatic stress disorder.

In this book, Martha focuses on what I believe is the most primal, terrifying, toxic, and motivating of all burdens: shame. Why is shame so powerful? Because when we feel shameful, we believe, at some level, that we are worthless. When we get the message in childhood that we are not treasured and loved by caretakers, we fear for our survival. Children are aware that their survival depends on being valuable to adults, and children who aren't valued die every day all over the world. So children—and adults, too—will do anything to distract from, counter, or otherwise avoid the fate of being shameful. As Martha writes in Chapter 3, "Children can bear bad things happening, but they don't know how to bear the idea that they are bad. When a child accepts global condemnation of their worth, they're doomed to go on and expend a preponderance of their psychic energy justifying and trying to validate their existence. Adults who come to therapy are still doing this—or their parts are doing it." Consider, for example, what depression, anxiety, unstable relational patterns, eating disorders, substance use problems, and other addictive processes such as overuse of pornography, gambling, and compulsive sexual risk taking all have in common. Martha argues convincingly that shame or guilt are often at the heart of these problems and that therapy won't be completely successful until those burdens are unloaded.

Unpacking shame as a relational phenomenon, inside and out, she describes a self-perpetuating shame cycle. A vulnerable part is shamed. Proactive protectors try to improve or hide that part with more shaming. The vulnerable part feels worse. Reactive protectors resort to extreme behaviors to avoid that feeling of shamefulness. Their behaviors evoke more shaming by external others and also ongoing accusations about weakness, lack of willpower, and harm to others by those proactive managerial protectors inside. Their shaming, in turn, increases the vulnerable part's sense of worthlessness and unlovability and motivates more extreme reactive behavior, and so it goes. Meanwhile, proactive protectors shame us for other reasons as well. They want us to look perfect, perform at a high level, or, conversely, act small to avoid risks. They will trigger the sense of worthlessness deliberately so that we will try harder or withdraw more. In this way, protectors are constantly using shame as a tool to keep us safe.

Guilt is another matter, and Martha clarifies the crucial differences between shame and guilt, as well as between adaptive and maladaptive guilt. After explaining and illustrating her nonpathologizing, empowering take on guilt and shame in the first half of the book, Martha tells us how we can heal from them in the second half. I'm happy and proud to report that her answer is IFS. To illustrate her points, she offers lucid case examples and experiential exercises that are tailored for resolving guilt and unburdening shame and that add nuance and insight to the basics of IFS. Martha's beautiful explanations and illustrations show readers that IFS is well equipped to address these supercharged burdens. I'm grateful. And I'll add that, as shame is a topic of global interest and IFS has become a global movement, I hope this book will grace the shelves of readers and thinkers all over the world.

RICHARD C. SCHWARTZ, PhD
Developer of the IFS model
Adjunct Faculty, Department of Psychiatry,
Harvard Medical School

Preface

How This Book Can Simplify Your Job

First, some things you don't have to worry about.

The client changing.

In therapy, clients don't need to be anywhere else or change who they are. They need to access resources that will make their bodies and minds habitable.

Knowing more about your client than your client.

You are equipped to ask the right kind of questions (open-ended, focused on motivation), and you can count on some part of the client having the relevant information to share when it's ready and willing.

Giving advice.

In some situations, it may feel right to give advice—for example, if you have some information the client doesn't have, or if they're engaging in a dangerous behavior, such as fighting with their partner while one of them is driving a car, driving after drinking alcohol, or having risky, unprotected sex. But, in general, if a client needs to solve a problem, you can listen to their internal viewpoints and facilitate what I call *unblending*, which I explain and illustrate at length in this book.

Hard work.

Manager parts work hard, and therapist parts are hardworking managers. If you find yourself working, you may be siding with a client's manager part and aggravating internal tensions. I'll say more about all that later on. It's more effective, as I illustrate, to be curious.

Summary Boxes and Exercises for You and Your Clients

Readers will find summary boxes and topic-specific exercises throughout. These can be photocopied or used as prompts for writing in a journal or on handy note paper.

How This Book Can Help You Do Your Job

Readers will learn to

- Address resistance effectively.
- Use hypotheticals to avoid power struggles that lead to therapeutic impasse.
- Redirect projections and guide safe internal inquiry.
- Promote kind internal relationships.
- Rescript traumatic experiences that leave the client feeling stuck in the past.
- Help clients be self-aware and practice self-compassion on a regular basis.

If these options interest you, read on.

Acknowledgments

I thank, as always, my lifelong partner (we went to grade school together), Rob Postel, for his exceptional patience and support. I thank my clients who have taught me, generally with patience and good humor, how to be of help. I thank my friends Colleen Gillard and Sandy Wells for giving me pointers on how to write for publication many years ago. I started in the field of mental health in 1987, and this book is the sum of everything I've learned. I thank my dissertation advisor, Bob Shilkret, who introduced me to Control Mastery theory, and Professor Gerry Schamess, now gone, for his open heart, wisdom, good humor, and gift for listening. I thank the many remarkable teachers and colleagues I've learned from and with over many years. I'll mention just a few by name, starting with my smart, generous, kind colleagues from the Cambridge Health Alliance (CHA): Matt Leeds (whom I also thank for reading this book and making valuable suggestions), Janna Smith, Nancy Blum, Nan Hellman, Wes Boyd, Linda Hutton, Karsten Kueppenbender, and, though they're gone now, Nina Masters and Les Havens. For the good company and good times learning Affect Phobia therapy, I thank Nat Kuhn and my fellow learners (in alphabetical order) Emily Bailey, Vida Kazemi, Jan Weathers, and Liz Zoob. For their support of Internal Family Systems (IFS) therapy at CHA, I thank Jay Burke and Michael Williams. For their generous willingness to be on the team and teach IFS therapy at the CHA, either briefly or over the course of many years, I thank (in alphabetical order) the following: Jim Abrams, Carita Anderson, Melissa Coco, Mike Elkin, Fatimah Finney, Gail Hardenberg, Deb Haynor, Nicole Herschenhous, Lance Hicks, Priscilla Howell, Bridge Kiley, Norma Kisaiti, Mary Kruger, Barbara Levine, Dave Lovas, Paul

Neustadt, Brian Orr, Vanessa Peavy, Andrew Prokopis, Danielle Schuman-Olivier, Gary Simoneau, Hanna Soumerai, Leah Soumerai, Jill Stanzler-Katz, Joyce Sullivan, Mary Catherine Ward, and Annie Weiss. I thank Toni Herbine-Blank, Anne Hallward, and Gary Whited, the three who presented a preconference day with me a few years ago on the topic of shame. I thank my Cambridge Hospital IFS research mates (in alphabetical order) Larry Rosenberg, Zev Schuman-Olivier, Dick Schwartz, Nancy Sowell, Hanna Soumerai, and Mary Catherine Ward. I thank Toni Herbine-Blank, Jory Agate, and Morgan Lindsey—my Shame Camp compatriots. I am always grateful to Dick Schwartz, the founder of IFS. Finally, a bow to the team at The Guilford Press. I'm grateful to Jane Keislar for her work on the manuscript; Elaine Kehoe for her help with copyediting; Laura Specht Patchkofsky for overseeing the book to its final form; Paul Gordon for the beautiful cover design; and Jim Nageotte, my editor, for his skillful guidance and warm, kind encouragement. Without his interest, this book would not be.

Contents

INTERNAL FAMILY SYSTEMS THERAPY
FOR SHAME AND GUILT

Introduction

The more scientists dig into life—microbes, plants, invertebrates, vertebrates—the more they find systems and systems within systems. Recent findings on the human gut, for example, show bacteria, fungi, and parasites in the trillions living with us symbiotically and serving crucial functions. Human beings also create and participate in interdependent external systems such as families, work environments, schools, and places of worship. In addition to these physiological and external systems, our psyche hosts a complex social system. The premise of this book is that the psyche's social system includes numerous separate centers of motivation (or, more colloquially, *parts*) with different points of view who communicate by way of feelings, sensations, and thoughts. In this light, we can understand the aftermath of trauma as a systemic response that brings many perspectives to the overriding goal of safety.

For our purposes, the word *trauma* covers a broad spectrum of relational experience, including everything from extremes that are obviously traumatic (childhood neglect, physical or sexual abuse, rape, war) to private experiences of invalidation, which others either might not notice or might not credit as formative. Whether intentional or not, trauma delivers the message that we're unworthy and unacceptable. Once we agree, the problem is all ours. This book explores how shame in action inside the mind (shaming) transforms this kind of injury into an identity (the state of being shameful) and how to remedy this problem using Internal Family Systems (IFS) therapy, which Richard Schwartz developed late in the 20th century based on the idea that the psyche is a system of independently motivated entities, or parts (Schwartz & Sweezy, 2020).

The idea of the plural mind dates far back in the field of mental health and is not original to IFS. I would even say the whole project of psychotherapy relies on the concept of more than one manifestation of consciousness—of the client being an observer as well as the observed. Sigmund Freud noticed psychic conflict and proposed three different minds, the *I* (ego), the *it* (id), and the *above-I* (superego). He was working in the late 19th century. Decades later, Marsha Linehan (1993), who developed dialectical behavior therapy (DBT), proposed an alternate model of three minds: *emotion mind*, *reasonable mind*, and *wise mind*. Many pioneers in the field of mental health who came along between these two clinicians conceived of a less aggregated, abstract plural mind, more along the lines of the model Schwartz developed, including Roberto Assagioli (1993), Carl Jung (1969), Fritz Perls and colleagues (1951), Helen and Jon Watkins (1997), and Hal and Sidra Stone (1993).

Schwartz came to his view of the mind pragmatically, while working as a family therapist. Sticking close to his clients' subjective experiences, he veered from orthodox family therapy views to develop a plural model of mind. In this model, it's normal for a person to have what his clients called *parts*. By listening to them, Schwartz found that parts are like people. They have motives, feelings, and opinions and take on different roles within their system. His clients also spoke of their *Self* to describe a distinct phenomenon of consciousness that differed from parts. In print, he chose the uppercase *S* to distinguish this form of consciousness as universal, in contrast to the lowercase-*s* self that signifies personal identity. In a balanced system, the Self leads the (theoretically infinite) community of parts. When this arrangement is disturbed, we suffer.

Previous mental health trailblazers had also described a unique form of consciousness. Both Freud and Linehan proposed a self-observant, self-monitoring inner leader. Freud's "above-I" (superego) was forbiddingly Victorian in comparison with Linehan's "wise mind" (on loan from Buddhism), but both were posed as a universal resource that offered a bird's-eye view of human affairs, just like the Self in IFS. After discovering the good effects of having access to this resource, Schwartz went to the library and discovered that all contemplative spiritual practices name some facsimile for the same concept. To mention just a few, in Buddhism it is Buddha mind, in Hinduism it is Atman, in Sufism it is the Beloved, and in Quakerism it is the Inner Light (Schwartz & Falconer, 2017).

I wrote this book because I wanted to spell out the ways in which therapy that is based on the concept of a plural mind led me to numerous interactions with clients that challenged all of my prior assumptions about human motivation and behavior. Although I work with adults, I gradually came to the conclusion that my most important customers in therapy were children—younger iterations of the person sitting in front of me—and I talk a lot about child parts in this book. Although others have written about IFS therapy with children (Johnson & Schwartz, 2000; Krause, 2013; Mones, 2014; Spiegel, 2017), in this book we look at the child parts of adults. In the chapters to come, I show how we can heal from shame-related identity injuries and release young parts from burdened bonds using treatment strategies that any mental health practitioner can learn to use. You need not be trained in IFS to understand my examples or follow my argument.

SECTION I

The Vulnerable Mind

In this first section, I employ numerous scenes from therapy to illustrate a number of assertions about the mind and how it functions. Whether you agree with these assertions or not, I hope they—along with my illustrations—will capture your attention and enrich your own explorations.

CHAPTER 1

Shame, Guilt, and Psychic Multiplicity

People generally come through bad experiences with an important question: *Why did this happen to me?* They also have answers. Accordingly, I ask them to listen to what they're hearing inside. Here is an example. Josie was a 30-year-old, cisgender, asexual, German-English American woman. An only child, she had gone through extreme trauma in childhood with her ferociously ambitious parents, who were revered leaders in their church and town. Josie's mother, for example, attached her to a leash that led to a pole in the living room and forced her to spend hours practicing the violin after school and on weekends. If no one was nearby to release her, she went hungry and might urinate on herself. If Josie broke one of her mother's arbitrary rules, she was left in the basement overnight to sleep on the floor. If she complained to her father, he hit her. She was not allowed to play with other children, watch television, or participate in sports. As expected, Josie attended a prestigious college and got into medical school, but she was unable to function there or in a workplace. She could not relate to peers or any person of authority. By the age of 27, she was living alone on disability in subsidized housing. At the time of this exchange, she had been in therapy just a few months.

● Josie Asks Why

JOSIE: Why me?

THERAPIST: What do you hear when you ask that question?

JOSIE: I'm bad.

7

THERAPIST: One part of you wonders, *Why me?* and another part replies, *You're bad.*

JOSIE: Isn't it true?

THERAPIST: What do you hear?

JOSIE: If you think you're getting out of this, you little bitch, think again!

If Josie heard something kinder when she wondered why her parents had tortured her, she would have needed less therapy. But her protective parts were as venomous as her parents. If I had challenged them by saying positive things about Josie, they would have tried to neutralize my interference. Positive assertions, inside or out, require a receptive audience. As long as protectors remain at odds with each other and don't know or trust the Self, they will veto hope and optimism vigorously. That doesn't stop me from being optimistic out loud about a client's prospects, but I don't argue. Rather, I praise the good intentions and hard work of their protectors and suggest that their reasons for being pessimistic were completely valid in the past. Then I ask if they are willing to be scientists. *Be skeptical,* I say, *but experiment. Hold us to a rigorous standard of honesty regarding results and try something new.*

As you will notice in this book, I speak with parts the way I speak with people. In that parts feel, think, and take on different roles in relation to each other, they are like people. At the same time, they're not like people. They can transform at will, shift shape, appear and disappear, expand and contract. Their environment, the psyche, is not like the material environment. It is a nonmaterial multiverse that has no physical constraints. Although we often find parts in the body, they can also be outside the body. Their moment-to-moment transformations are the stuff of science fiction, fantasy novels, and the untamed imagination. And, of course, they routinely travel through time.

Perhaps most important for our purposes, a part can take over mentally and make us see the world through its eyes. Internal Family Systems (IFS) therapy calls this *blending.* Bossy protective parts will take over, or blend, and say *I am you* to the client. The irony of having to insist *I am you* is lost on the part. But if it isn't *me,* who is? When the blended part separates—or differentiates—both from other parts and from the Self (which IFS calls *unblending*), we suddenly see the world—and our parts—very differently. This is when clients speak of feeling as if they are now *the real me, the true me,* and so on. How much separation (by report from the client) is required to get this effect? Thirty percent seems sufficient, but 50% (or more) is better. The *me* who shows up when parts separate is the Self, which doesn't feel like a part or even like all parts combined. The Self is a different manifestation of consciousness, an overarching phenomenon that exists outside of and beyond parts. Because the level of blending by parts governs the client's access to their Self, we can gauge both by asking, *Out of 100%, how blended is this part?* A specific number usually pops into the client's head.

We explore the concept of unblending at length in the chapters to come because it's crucial to therapeutic success. For now, I'll just say that some people view the brain as a receiver of various forms of consciousness, and I'm among them. But readers need not share this view. You can understand the concepts presented in this book, hear from your parts, and experience your Self without adhering to any particular theory about what's going on. We all bring our beliefs about what we don't know—and about what no one knows—to our experience. In any case, we are going to focus on exploring the roles of shame and guilt in psychic distress, starting from the premise that the mind is plural and includes this phenomenon we're calling the Self.

Shame and guilt are called the *self-conscious emotions.* Both feelings involve someone inside observing and blaming—shaming or guilting—and someone else inside feeling shameful or guilty. For a number of reasons, young children are exceptionally vulnerable to being shamed or guilted by external others. For one thing, they are radically innocent. Every experience is new and open to interpretation once. For another, they are completely dependent and highly attuned to adult caretakers. Shaming, which picks on specific characteristics of behavior or appearance, is news—bad news—for a child's internal system about a member of the internal community or some feature of the body. When either a part or the body is shamed, other parts, who are often the same age or just slightly older, galvanize for action. They may report having sensed that something fundamental at the child's core was under attack. They may say, for example, that the openhearted child invites predation, the curious child gets reprimanded, the brave one is a threat, the loud one is too much, the joyful one provokes censure, the compassionate one evokes fear, and the one who is unwanted must hide. Schwartz learned that some protective parts are intrepid first responders. They aim to protect the injured part. I follow his lead by calling them *managers.*

Ironically, managers favor responding to shaming with shaming. To improve, inhibit, or hide the part who drew fire, manager parts tend to take authority by incorporating the shamer's actions, thoughts, and feelings and becoming copycat shamers. Their shaming tends to be intentional, compulsive, and repetitive. They instruct the child, "*Do* be this; *don't* be that." They judge, admonish, frighten, and intimidate, or they overprotect and smother as a way of silencing. At either extreme, they drive vulnerable parts under rocks, up canyons, into cages, behind walls, and out of awareness. Following Schwartz again, I call these banished parts *exiles.*

All this shaming and condemnation by inner critics shocks the autonomic nervous system and scares the exiled parts, who feel shameful. In response, a second set of responders comes online to deflect, distract, soothe, and counteract their harshness. Schwartz called these parts *firefighters*. They are reactive protectors and, depending on what works best in the moment, they have many tactics to choose among. When less extreme, they focus on counterbalancing *shoulds* with *wants*. Take a break! Ride your bike, read, swim, paint a picture, play a game, sleep on the beach. Do something for the fun of it. But in extremity, firefighter parts will lead a person to drink, use drugs, have risky sex, look at porn compulsively, gamble, binge on sweets and fats, get mad, live in a virtual world, and so on. Along with a dismissive disregard for long-term consequences, their shameless, compulsive, impulsive behavior makes them look irrational. But in truth they're just as goal-driven as shaming managers. Their activities signal that the managerial project has failed.

The Road to Psychotherapy
Is Paved with Impossible Responsibilities and Blame

When a client tells their story at the outset of therapy, I listen for shaming and guilting, shamefulness and guiltiness. Here are four examples that illustrate a range of possibilities.

● Mona: Jealousy, Adaptive Guilt, and Shaming

Mona, a 34-year-old, cisgender, heterosexual, single, Czech American woman came to see me when she found herself envying her 4-year-old daughter, Mia. This envy began when Mona's mother, Marlee, offered to take care of Mia while Mona went back to work as a lawyer. Because Marlee had been cold and critical when she was a child, Mona was reluctant to accept her help. But she had to earn money, and Mia seemed delighted with the idea. So she accepted Marlee's help. As the arrangement succeeded over the next few months, Mona felt increasingly excluded and resentful of her daughter as well as her mother.

MONA: What kind of person begrudges a little kid some fun?
THERAPIST: What do you hear inside when you ask that question?
MONA: A bad mother. A monster.

Inner critics were guilting and shaming her: *You DO wrong* (guilting—refers to an action), *so you ARE bad* (shaming—refers to a state of being). This inner diatribe brought Mona to therapy. It was a good starting point for our exploration. To orient Mona to the idea of parts, I cited this inner shaming. We can always start therapy safely with critical managers. They like to be noticed, and they want to go first. From my perspective, Mona's guilt was adaptive because it warned her that she could harm her child emotionally if her jealous part stayed in control. This was an appropriate concern. However, the shaming (*you are bad*) was not adaptive. On the contrary, the shaming sparked a countervailing resentment and urge to blame her daughter, which reactivated her guilt and made it hard for her to seek help.

● Alex: Not Belonging and Self-Shaming

Here is another example, this one involving shamefulness without guilt. Alex, a nonbinary, asexual, Asian American, came to therapy at 25 after years of crippling social anxiety. From grade school through college, sensory integration issues had caused Alex to shy away from groups of kids.

THERAPIST: What brings you to therapy?

ALEX: (*Shrugs.*) I'm lonely.

THERAPIST: Say more.

ALEX: I don't belong. I never have.

THERAPIST: Can you give me an example?

ALEX: When I moved here for a job last fall, I wanted to find roommates. But I just couldn't imagine that working out. So I'm living alone and spending most of my salary on rent.

THERAPIST: One part of you wanted to live with other people, but another part told you that couldn't work, is that right?

ALEX: Yes.

THERAPIST: What, specifically, do you hear about why it can't work?

ALEX: *Everyone despises you in the end.*

When other people were relaxing and having fun, Alex was shy and avoidant because their nervous system was painfully overstimulated. In response, some people (though not all) felt shunned and responded in kind. While Alex had parts who longed to be included socially and have friends, they also had a shaming part who wanted to keep them from reaching out and getting rejected. As we discovered over time, Alex was depressed as well as anxious. Their anxiety was the product of forward-looking protection (*you will be rejected*), and their sense of oppression and depression were the product of backward-looking shaming (*I have always been different and inadequate*). For Alex, anxiety and depression were a package deal.

● Sharon: Impossible Choices and Maladaptive Guilt

Sharon had to make a decision but had a reasonable expectation that either choice would lead to bad consequences. As a result, she felt guilty in advance of choosing. As you read about her dilemma, ask yourself if her guilt was adaptive or maladaptive. She was a 20-year-old, cisgender, heterosexual, Guatemalan American college student who had come to the United States from Guatemala at the age of 2 with her undocumented parents. Just as she began college, her parents were both deported back to Guatemala. Because she qualified as a "Dreamer," she was able to stay and continue in school. Then her father had a stroke.

SHARON: I'm so afraid for my parents. I don't know what to do.

THERAPIST: What are your options?

SHARON: I could go to Guatemala. I grew up in Minneapolis. I don't know what kind of job I could get. I haven't finished college, and my Spanish is childish. If I go, I could never come back. I'd be in a foreign country permanently. I was planning to help them with money after college. But how can they be alone now? I don't know what to do.

THERAPIST: I hear this is a huge dilemma. Your parents need help and you want to be with them, but the cost of leaving the United States would be tremendous, possibly for them as well as you.

SHARON: I don't know what to do. I don't want to regret this decision, but no matter what I do, I think I will.

Sharon has no internal conflict over her relationship with her parents. She wants to protect them. She is comfortable with the idea of making sacrifices for them, but she doesn't know which sacrifice to make. Stay in the United States and hope they will survive long enough for her to send them money once she is working? Or leave to take care of them with scant means to earn money? Fearing harm to all of them, she feels guilty in advance of either decision. Because her guilt is understandable but not deserved, it is maladaptive. Though she—and her parents—have much to lose either way, her choice, whatever it is, will not be a transgression.

● Harley: Parentification and Maladaptive Guilt

In this example the maladaptive guilt is easy to spot. Harley, a 20-year-old, cisgender, heterosexual, English American, was gifted in computer science but was stalled professionally and personally after a difficult childhood. His younger brother had died of brain cancer when he was 12. After his death, Harley's father had spent more time at work and had started drinking with friends after work and on weekends. His mother had become chronically depressed and spent much of the day in a darkened bedroom. When he was 17, Harley's father drove off a bridge and drowned. Although the police ruled it a drunk driving accident, Harley thought it was suicide. His school counselor, who knew his mother was financially stable and had relatives nearby, urged him to apply to competitive colleges around the country and wanted him to accept when he was offered a good scholarship. Instead, Harley stayed home, went to a nearby community college with no scholarship, and worked while taking night classes. And at the end of 2 years, he got a full-time job as a computer tech in a large company. He came to therapy because his cousin was pressing him to reconsider finishing college.

HARLEY'S RESPONSIBLE MANAGER: I'm only here because Michael insisted. I didn't want to disappoint him.

THERAPIST: You didn't want to disappoint him?

HARLEY'S RESPONSIBLE MANAGER: I don't like to disappoint people.

THERAPIST: What does Michael say?

HARLEY'S RESPONSIBLE MANAGER: He thinks I should finish college.

THERAPIST: You don't want to finish college?

HARLEY'S RESPONSIBLE MANAGER: No. I'd like to finish college. But I got a job.

THERAPIST: So, one part of you would like to finish college, but another part wanted to get a job?

HARLEY'S RESPONSIBLE MANAGER: I thought I should get a job.

THERAPIST: Another part thought you should get a job instead of finishing college.

HARLEY'S RESPONSIBLE MANAGER: Yes.

THERAPIST: So, this is an internal argument? (*Harley nods noncommittally.*) And Michael agrees with the part who thinks you should finish college.

HARLEY: I guess so.

THERAPIST: What would the other part, the one who wants you to have a job, be concerned about if you finished college instead?

HARLEY'S RESPONSIBLE MANAGER: Nothing.

[*This answer is an evasion, probably by the guilty manager part who caused him to stay home and get a job.*]

THERAPIST: Let's talk with both these parts.

[*When in doubt, convene a meeting.*]

HARLEY: Okay.

THERAPIST: Can you see them?

HARLEY: Yeah, sort of. They're just two shadows standing a few feet apart.

THERAPIST: Which of them needs your attention first?

HARLEY: The one who wants to stay home is louder.

THERAPIST: Stay home means keep your current job? (*Harley nods.*) How do you feel toward that part?

[*This* Geiger-counter *question, as I call it, measures Self-energy.*]

HARLEY'S REBELLIOUS PART: I'm tired of him.

THERAPIST: Would the part or parts who are tired of him be willing to step back so you can talk with him?

HARLEY: That's a funny idea.

THERAPIST: Isn't it? See if they'll do it.

HARLEY: Okay.

THERAPIST: How do you feel toward him now?

HARLEY'S REBELLIOUS PART: I wish he'd go away.

THERAPIST: Could I talk with him while you listen? (*Harley nods.*) Just let him talk through your mouth. I want to talk with the part who wants Harley to keep the job. Are you there?

HARLEY'S RESPONSIBLE MANAGER: Yes.

THERAPIST: What are you concerned would happen to Harley if he went to college?

HARLEY'S RESPONSIBLE MANAGER: He'd never come back.

THERAPIST: And what would be the problem with that?

HARLEY'S RESPONSIBLE MANAGER: She'd kill herself.

THERAPIST: Who?

HARLEY'S RESPONSIBLE MANAGER: His mother.

THERAPIST: She said that?

HARLEY'S RESPONSIBLE MANAGER: Yes.

THERAPIST: And then what would happen?

HARLEY'S RESPONSIBLE MANAGER: He'd be responsible.

THERAPIST: I see. I'm going to talk with Harley again, okay? (*Harley nods.*) Did you hear that, Harley?

HARLEY: Yes.

THERAPIST: How do you feel toward this part now?

HARLEY: (*Sighs.*) That's why I'm tired.

THERAPIST: I understand. This part is worried and loud. And I bet the other part, the one who wants you to go to college, is also worried. What if we could help these parts so you could decide how to proceed?

HARLEY: Me?

THERAPIST: Yes. You. The Harley-who's-not-a-part.

HARLEY'S RESPONSIBLE MANAGER: I don't know how to help anyone.

THERAPIST: I know you feel that way now. This will help—if everyone is willing. Take a minute and listen inside.

HARLEY: Okay.

Real as the possibility may have been that Harley's mother would act on her suicide threats (I had no way of assessing that), staying home with her was not his only option. He could talk with her about getting help, attend therapy with her, and generally take steps to prepare her so that he could pursue his own life. His anticipatory guilt—the warnings of a protective manager part—about the way she might react was maladaptive because pursuing normal developmental goals is not a transgression.

Shame and Guilt

The self-conscious emotions, shame and guilt, both generate negative self-referential judgments. Nonetheless, as Helen Block Lewis (1971), June Tangney and Rhonda Dearing (2002), Judith Lewis Herman (2015), and others have explained, we shouldn't conflate the two. Guilt involves an assessment of behavior (*I did wrong*), whereas shame is a global assessment of value (*I am . . . unworthy, defective, unlovable*, etc.). Guilt generates concern for the injured other, along with the urge to repair the relationship. In contrast, shame—signifying an internal process in which one part does some shaming and another part feels shameful—leads to fear, hiding, and (reactively) rage. Feeling guilty about one's behavior toward someone else and shaming oneself lead us in different directions.

Guilt

If I do something hurtful, I have transgressed, and guilt helps me to be active about approaching the other person and making a repair. We all transgress at times, more or less egregiously, and guilt is the appropriate and adaptive (positive, constructive, reconnecting, growth-producing) response. It walks us back from thoughtless stumbles, isolating, self-interested behavior, and worse. But we don't have to transgress to feel guilty. As the preceding examples illustrate, guilt can be maladaptive. For example, it can develop from relational loyalty. Separation and survivor guilt are the prime examples of maladaptive guilt. As we see with Harley, a high school graduate might feel guilty about leaving a parent with depression to go to college. Underlying this decision, the child has a separation guilt belief: *If I pursue my needs and wants, I will hurt this person for whom I am responsible.*

Survivor guilt involves a similar though slightly different underlying belief: *My gains and successes come at the expense of people I love or for whom I feel responsible.* We can see this in, for example, a successful person who remains chronically depressed despite circumstances that would normally produce optimism and pleasure. Unable to rescue their family, they have a part who stays connected, does penance, and feels morally redeemed by renouncing personal happiness. As with separation guilt, survivor guilt causes us to act as if our pursuit of positive personal goals is transgressive and, further, as if self-sacrifice is reparation. We generally benefit by being attuned to the feelings, views, and needs of others, but when we sacrifice personal goals to comfort, soothe, or take care of someone who is emotionally unavailable, inappropriately dependent, or literally dead, guilt is a problem.

Shame

I suggest thinking of shame as an act (*shaming*) or a state of being (*shameful*). When we shame, we judge another person globally on the basis of a particular behavior, quality, or feature of their body, culture, or life circumstance. Condemning the whole for a part gives shaming its harsh, blunt impact. Rather than charging *You did . . .* (something hurtful), shaming alleges *You are . . .* (bad, defective, too much, too little, etc.). If we *do* something wrong, we can at least make an effort at repair, but if we *are* defective, there is no escape. When a condemned part is taken to represent a whole system, the obvious solution for that system is to differentiate from or improve the offending part.

We might see this, for example, in a person trying to conform more effectively, be more acceptable, wear different clothes, do things to appear taller or shorter, change their hair, lose weight, gain weight, change their face, change their accent, forswear ancestors, lose the family religion, move to a new zip code, accumulate things, give things away, be a star, be invisible, and generally try to become the opposite of whatever they were shamed for being. And this is what manager parts lead us to do. Ironically, their improvement efforts serve to reinforce the belief that the original shaming was accurate information.

Until recently, Western culture has not viewed individuals as systems. As a result, our identities tend to get defined by our vulnerabilities or strengths, and our protectors naturally prefer the latter. But if you think in terms of parts, it's easy to see that one part does not represent all parts. So, let's consider two questions. When someone inside is shaming, who is doing the shaming? And who has the power to challenge it? In answer to the first question, inner shamers are good mimics and are quick to learn from external others. Sometimes an external person shames inadvertently, sometimes intentionally.

In this book, we look at the effects of both. Some intentional shamers shame in the name of improving others. Parents and other authority figures who believe that shaming socializes children fall in this category, as do adults who shame other adults to police their behavior. We need only survey high-conflict couples or look at the Internet to notice how many adults believe that shaming will produce good, as in constructive and positive, results. But other shamers make no moral or educational excuse. They shame to (1) reboot their personal sense of value by feeling bigger, stronger, and more worthy than someone else; (2) exert control; (3) accrue power; or (4) profit materially—or some combination.

Whatever the shamer's intentions, the recipient of shaming will feel hurt but may not feel shameful. Let's pause to highlight this point: To feel shameful, we must believe the message. The continuum of receptivity to shaming runs from zero (the supremely self-confident individual who feels unassailable), to a bit vulnerable (the person who questions their worth for some particular reason, such as, e.g., a recent divorce), to the most vulnerable (say, a child or an adult who is financially dependent, or anyone who already feels worthless). We receive shaming according to our place on this continuum. At the most vulnerable end, we absorb shaming as confirmation of existing negative beliefs about who we are and what we're worth.

Receiving Shaming

The crucial point is that a shamed person will either accept shaming or decline to feel shameful, according to their vulnerability. Once a vulnerable person has accepted shaming, they're stuck with feeling shameful and are primed to believe any future shaming that comes their way. Furthermore, the recipient of shaming who feels shameful will eventually try to recoup their balance and distract from inner critics by shaming others, whether they recognize this or not.

EXERCISE

Differentiating Shame, Maladaptive Guilt, and Adaptive Guilt

1. **The Cognitions of Shame, Maladaptive Guilt, and Adaptive Guilt**
   - Shame: *I am bad* (defective, too much, too little, etc.).
   - Maladaptive guilt, due to a transgression, fused with shame: *I did wrong and I am bad.*
   - Maladaptive guilt, *not* due to a transgression, fused with shame: *I did wrong and I am bad.*
   - Adaptive, "pure" guilt, due to a transgression: *I did wrong and I need to make a repair.*

2. **Quiz Yourself: Is It Shame, Maladaptive Guilt, or Adaptive Guilt?** (Circle the ones that apply.)

   a. *I am bad:* (1) shame, (2) maladaptive guilt, (3) adaptive guilt

   b. The client did commit a transgression and believes *I did wrong and I am bad:* (1) shame, (2) maladaptive guilt, (3) adaptive guilt

   c. The client did not commit a transgression but still believes *I did wrong and I am bad:* (1) shame, (2) maladaptive guilt, (3) adaptive guilt

   d. The client did commit a transgression and believes *I did wrong and I need to make a repair:* (1) shame, (2) maladaptive guilt, (3) adaptive guilt

   [Key: a = 1, b = 3 + 1, c = 2 + 1, d = 3]

3. **Outcome Goals: Challenging Shame and Maladaptive Guilt**

   - Shame: I'm bad.
     - The Goal: *I'm fine.*
   - Guilt after a transgression that is fused with shame: *I did wrong so I am bad.*
     - The Goal: *I did wrong, I am not bad, I will repair the consequences.*
   - Guilt that is *not* due to a transgression but is fused with shame: *I did wrong and I am bad.*
     - The Goal: *I did not do wrong and I am not bad.*

Addressing the Shame Cycle

Shaming is a highly contagious behavior that infects relationships inside and out. All of us do some intrapsychic and interpersonal shaming at some point. So, where do we intervene?

Language

Let's start with language, which either obscures or illuminates what we'll be calling the *shame cycle*. When a client says, "I feel a lot of shame," I don't know if they're talking about a part who is being shamed or a part who is shaming. But I'll find out if I personify their experience with parts language and substitute the words *shaming* and *shameful* for *shame*. Here is an example.

● Raphael Feels Ashamed and Shames Himself

Raphael, a 35-year-old, cisgender, heterosexual, Argentinian American man, came to therapy after being dropped by his girlfriend because, when she proposed marriage, he felt compelled to say no even though he didn't want to end the relationship. This was his first session.

RAPHAEL: I feel a lot of shame.

THERAPIST: Want to explore that?

[*Ask for permission before diving in.*]

RAPHAEL: Yes.

THERAPIST: Is someone shaming you inside?

[*Although he uses the word* shame, *he could be thinking of a part who shames him or a part who feels shameful. Because it's likely to be a critic who shames him, I check for that first.*]

RAPHAEL: Yes, of course.

THERAPIST: How do you know it's there?

RAPHAEL: It's a voice. Not an out-loud kind of voice. It's in my head.

THERAPIST: Do you see anyone speaking?

RAPHAEL: Not right now.

THERAPIST: Have you ever talked to this voice?

RAPHAEL: No.

THERAPIST: How do you feel toward it?

RAPHAEL: Are you kidding? I hate it!

THERAPIST: Would it be okay to ask it a question?

RAPHAEL: (*Shrugs uncomfortably.*) Okay.

THERAPIST: Is it a part of you?

RAPHAEL: (*Gives me a worried, puzzled look.*) What do you mean?

[*We have not yet talked about the concept of parts.*]

THERAPIST: I will explain, but first, if this is okay with you, ask this inner shamer if it is a part of you.

[*I want to know if he experiences this voice as* me *or* not me. *If the answer is* not me, *I will talk with him about inherited burdens, as I discuss and illustrate in Chapters 6 and 7. If the answer is* me, *I will focus on helping him to befriend his critic—as illustrated below.*]

RAPHAEL: (*Closes his eyes and is quiet for a few beats.*) It's part of me.

[*Raphael gets an answer and has first contact with a part.*]

THERAPIST: This critic is one of your parts. We all have parts. Lots of them, actually. Right now, you notice a shaming part and another part—or maybe lots of other parts—who hate the shaming part.

RAPHAEL: Yes.

THERAPIST: Would they be willing to relax and let you learn more about the shamer?

RAPHAEL: I don't feel comfortable with him.

THERAPIST: Do you see him?

RAPHAEL: It's my fifth-grade English teacher, Mr. Herd. He hated me. (*A short silence.*) I hear him saying that I'm stupid and stubborn and don't deserve help. But it can't really be him because he knows private things about me. So, it must be me.

THERAPIST: This copy of Mr. Herd insults you but is really a part of you.

RAPHAEL: I couldn't spell and he just . . . I don't know why, he hated me. I think he picked on the kids he could pick on.

THERAPIST: Who does this Mr. Herd copy protect?

RAPHAEL: (*A long silence.*) Me. I'm the one with shame.

THERAPIST: You have a part who feels shameful.

[*This time I translate his word* shame *to* shameful.]

RAPHAEL: A part? It seems like me.

THERAPIST: Let's find out. Would the Mr. Herd part agree to let you talk with the one who feels shameful?

RAPHAEL: (*Shakes his head.*) He says absolutely no.

THERAPIST: What would happen if you learned more about the part who feels shameful?

[*Protective parts are always motivated by specific fears that were reasonable in the past but may no longer apply.*]

RAPHAEL: I'd give up.

THERAPIST: Does that make sense to you, Raphael?

RAPHAEL: I wanted to give up a lot. I almost ran away in fifth grade, but I didn't have the courage. Herd wasn't the only one who found me disappointing.

THERAPIST: So, the part who copies Mr. Herd controls a part who wanted to run away and escape disappointed people?

[*I name what sounds to me like an inner polarity between two protective parts.*]

RAPHAEL: Yes.

THERAPIST: How do you feel toward the copy part now?

RAPHAEL: He's shrinking.

THERAPIST: Oh?

RAPHAEL: (*A few beats.*) He's 10.

THERAPIST: How do you feel toward him?

RAPHAEL: He says giving up will make things worse.

THERAPIST: In what way?

RAPHAEL: My mother did everything on her own. She brought me to the

U.S. to escape my biological father when I was a baby and she was nineteen. She raised me and went to law school at the same time. She's very smart and she never understood why I did bad in some subjects but great in others. It didn't matter to her that I'm dyslexic.

[Note that although Raphael did well in some subjects, his critical part reflects the shaming attitudes of the adults around him.]

THERAPIST: What did she tell herself—and you—about that?

RAPHAEL: She believes in willpower. She really couldn't understand me. I asked if I could live with my grandparents in Argentina. She did want me to learn Spanish, but she was afraid of my father. When she finally said yes, my abuela got sick and died.

THERAPIST: What did your mother say to you about school?

RAPHAEL: That I wasn't trying hard enough.

THERAPIST: Does the 10-year-old who copies Mr. Herd see you right now?

RAPHAEL: No.

THERAPIST: Would he like to?

RAPHAEL: Okay, he's looking.

THERAPIST: How does he respond?

RAPHAEL: He looks sad.

THERAPIST: He protects the dyslexic boy? (*Raphael nods.*) If you could help that boy, would it be good for him?

RAPHAEL: Yes.

THERAPIST: And if he didn't have to shame the dyslexic boy anymore, what would he rather do?

RAPHAEL: Ride his bike.

This session revealed a nucleus of distressing experiences in Raphael's childhood involving shaming, shamefulness, and loneliness. By speaking of shame in two distinct ways, as an action (shaming) or a state of being (shamefulness), we were able to untangle his inner experience, in which a 10-year-old copycat protector was looking and acting like a rageful, shaming teacher to help a dyslexic boy. Once he had contact with Raphael's Self, the copycat began to unhook from being a critic. In this session, our job was to befriend him and get permission from him to help the shamed boy.

The Function of Being Shamed

There is none. It's a bad experience, which harms the recipient if they believe it.

The Function of Shaming

Externally (this shamer may be a proactive manager or a reactive fire-fighter):

1. To feel bigger, more significant, and more powerful in comparison to someone who feels smaller, less significant, and weaker.
2. To control and dominate.
3. To profit.

Internally (this shamer is a proactive manager):

1. To improve or banish the exile and protect the individual's familial/social connections.
2. To control firefighter parts.

How else might shaming serve the shamer?

Burdens: Personal and Inherited

Exiles have shaming personal beliefs, which they often experience as literal physical encumbrances. In IFS, we call these beliefs *burdens*. An exile may say it carries a backpack full of rocks, it may feel immersed in sludge, be encased in armor, or feel inhabited by mold, tentacles, a false organ, and so on. In contrast, protectors have jobs. Their jobs, which spring from fear and a sense of responsibility, are also burdensome. When a child's loyal protectors join with a caretaker to share the caretaker's burden, the child, in essence, inherits their caretaker's burden (Sinko, 2017). Inherited burdens differ from personal burdens in a few important ways. A personal burden—a shame-based belief—develops involuntarily from personal experience. In contrast, an inherited burden takes up residence when a child shoulders a caretaker's burden out of loyalty, proximity, dependency, fear, identification, empathy, and so on. The personal burden is a shameful identity; the inherited burden tends to signal a guilt-based relationship. To differentiate the two, as the chapters to come discuss both, I call the burdens that develop from personal experience *identity burdens* and the burdens that originated with others *relational burdens*. In Chapters 6 and 7, I show how *burdened bonds* cause children to shoulder relational burdens. For now, it's just important to know that exiled parts get exiled both because they have identity burdens—they feel shameful—and because other parts believe they are shameful.

What's Change Got to Do with Therapy?

Clients tend to start therapy either seeking change or dreading it and refusing to change. Manager parts are the ones who seek change; they want to change the essence of the exile and the behavior of firefighter parts. They work hard and they're tired. Firefighters, on the other hand, focus more narrowly on changing the arousal state of the autonomic nervous system whenever threatening beliefs (*I'm worthless, I'm unlovable*) evoke strong feelings. They work hard, too, although they rarely admit to being tired.

If clients come to therapy with any intent, it's usually the managerial intent to change. Their manager team tells them to become a better person. Be braver. Be stronger. Be more lovable. Get control of that uncontrolled disinhibition. These parts expect the therapist to rally to the cause and lead them to success. If we focus on change in therapy, we reinforce their belief that self-reinvention can solve the problem of having been shamed, which it cannot. When we call therapy work (though I admit it can be hard to avoid the word), we inadvertently reinforce the managerial belief that working harder will change that shameful exile into someone lovable.

Because managerial efforts to change the exile are, from my perspective, at the heart of the problem, I don't want managers focusing on work or change in therapy. I interrupt work monologues (characterized by the word *do—What should I do? I have to do something. I try to do* this or that) to suggest that something different and better will happen if they stop working—in fact, they could stop right now and do nothing for a just few moments to see how it feels. I may joke about child labor laws, and I may say, in all seriousness, that I don't plan to work. Hard work won't help parts feel legitimate and lovable, and none of them needs to change who they are.

That said, my challenge to the ethos of earned love is certain to lack credibility at first. I know the client's Self can sanction a part's existence. I know the Self can annul harsh judgments. I know their exiles could see shamefulness as inaccurate information from a disturbed source and let it go. I know the whole internal system would be relieved if this were to happen. And I know that all parts need to be in relationship with the client's Self. Protectors don't have to *do* anything about this beyond being willing to stop doing whatever they do. When they stop doing and stand by, the Self shows up, which drains their drive to keep doing. But if this is to happen, they need direct experience with the Self. We may need to start with little experiments before protectors will allow bigger ones, but, in any case, change happens when protectors stop working on change.* When exiles

---

* As Carl Rogers said, "The curious paradox is that when *I accept myself, just* as *I* am, then *I can change.*"

unburden, protectors volunteer to open the sluice gates, life flows, and the normal state of things reasserts itself. The normal state of things is change.

A Model of Mind

If you endorse the idea of psychic multiplicity, it applies to everyone. That said, not everyone will want to interact with their parts or use this approach in therapy. Parts have to be willing to participate, and sometimes they're not. If a person comes to me expressing reluctance to talk about parts, I assume that a part is speaking, and I can only be curious about its concerns. If the client expresses some willingness to proceed despite their reluctant part, we can go on. I'm willing to use other words for parts. If they prefer to talk about feelings, sensations, thoughts, and so on, I can do that. But I make it clear that I think of feelings, sensations, and thoughts as the expressions and communications of parts. I tell clients that, as far as I'm concerned, the psyche is, by evolutionary design, a meeting place for the many opinions and perspectives of their parts. If they have no interest in this way of thinking, I can point them toward other resources.

　　If a client is willing to try my approach but their mind seems paralyzed or races, we'll think about adjunctive treatments, such as neurofeedback, medication (including ketamine and, down the road, I hope, MDMA and psilocybin), movement (yoga, dance), and so on, with an eye to what appeals and what the client can afford. But, in any case, sometimes protectors aren't willing to participate in therapy. All we can do is invite, offer, and, if at least some of the client's parts want, persist. We don't control parts. That said, when they believe the therapist understands how the inner system functions and knows how to maintain a baseline of safety, they're often eager to give this approach a try.

Conclusion

What we believe about shame and guilt matters a lot in therapy because most clients are struggling with one or both. I've said that shame is either *shaming*, a transgressive act of diminishment, or *shamefulness*, a simmering, poisoned state of being that gives rise to continual anxiety about one's legitimacy and value. Guilt, in contrast, is how one responds to having transgressed or having thought of transgressing. It signals relational concern. I am concerned for you because of what I've done (or might do) to you. Shaming is a transgressive act; guilt is a response (sometimes a proactive response) to acting transgressively. But they can intertwine. If an inner critic shames a guilty protector (*You did wrong so you're bad*), its shaming is likely to eclipse the feeling of guilt. As far as relationships go, it's far better for me to feel guilty than ashamed. Conscience guides repair. It's hardwired. We need to trust that. The best way to access our conscience is to calm inner shaming and be accountable.

Of course, some transgressions can't be repaired directly (because, e.g., the victim is dead or the transgressor doesn't have access to the victim for some reason). Then either the transgressor or their community have to fashion a repair that attempts to match the loss they caused and mend the social fabric they tore. Irreparable guilt can devolve due to shaming and become a kind of cognitive superglue (*This can never be fixed!*) for the feeling of shamefulness. In this case, only the transgressor or their community can judge when (if ever) their debt is discharged, as in the different but equally complex and imperfect South African, Rwandan, and Canadian reconciliation processes (Government of Canada, 2015; Mustafa, 2020; Weilanga, 2017). If no communal process exists to set an endpoint for guilt, reparations can go off track (as I show in Chapter 12) or may be a lifelong project. But we are equipped to address guilt. Transgressions require repair. Shaming and shamefulness interfere with the reparative workings of deserved guilt.

CHAPTER 2

The Goal

I've said the psyche consists of a community of parts and a contrasting resource, the Self. Philosophers call this arrangement *a unity of opposites*: without light we wouldn't have (or even need the concept of) darkness because we would only know darkness. Without death we would not have a concept of life, and so on. Pairs of opposites define each other. The Self and parts are such a pair. The idea that there is more than one form of consciousness is not new. Buddhists call the same resource *Buddha mind*; and Patanjali, the presumed author of ancient Sanskrit yoga sutras, wrote (as translated by Gregor Maehle, 2006, p. 200): *The seer is consciousness . . . which is awareness* [in IFS terms, the Self]. *The seen is not only the entire world of objects but also the inner instrument . . . consisting of intellect, mind, and ego* [in IFS terms, parts].* The ultimate success of IFS depends on clients and therapists accessing both forms of consciousness. When our parts make room for the Self, we feel mentally spacious, compassionate, and able to be curious rather than reactive. We have a bird's-eye view of ourselves, other people, and events. This is the goal of IFS therapy.

Parts can make room for the Self to show up, but they have to be willing. It's ironic, but the Self, which is always available to help out and take responsibility, doesn't control parts. We can't make our parts separate, and we don't do the separating for them. They have to cooperate. Sometimes they seem to be captive to the body and need assistance in the form of

---

*Thanks to IFS therapist and yoga teacher Allison Miller for sending me this Patanjali quote.

something like movement, neurofeedback, medication, and so on. But in any case, we can't order them around or trick them into quitting their jobs. Their willingness to stop doing and follow the Self's lead is as essential as the noncontrolling, inviting attitude of the Self. Willingness is therefore our first order of business. The Self earns the willingness of protectors by being inclusive, attentive, and interested. Until the client's Self is available to give that kind of attention, the therapist's Self stands in, as I illustrate in this chapter.

Accordingly, IFS devotes the first portion of therapy to the willingness of protective parts and the second to the needs and wishes of exiled parts. These distinct portions of therapy rarely require the same amount of time, with protectors needing the lion's share of attention. Some protectors will have had a bad experience of therapy in the past, some will fear being exposed and shamed now, some will have felt pressured to come to therapy, some will be terrified of emotional flooding if the client were to revisit traumatic events, some won't trust anyone. As well, most protectors endorse the status quo. They may not be happy with it, but they do believe something really is wrong with the vulnerable parts they exile. They believe the past predicts the future. They may believe they are responsible for the welfare of a caretaker, sibling, or other relative. They're afraid of not doing what they do. They need our persistent patience. When they're willing to unblend and test our assertion that the Self exists and exiles can be helped, we move on to the next portion of therapy.

In the second portion, the client's Self becomes the exile's audience and primary attachment figure. The exile may show details of its traumatic experiences to the Self, which the client usually reports to the therapist. Some exiles, however, don't feel the need to go into detail, and some don't want to share their story with anyone but the client's Self. The therapist is there as an additional witness as needed. The exile directs. As with the first portion of therapy, the essential therapeutic ingredients in this portion are curiosity and compassion. The following example, which occurred during an intake evaluation at a hospital, illustrates how I might help a client access their Self. Within 90 minutes, I was able to get basic information for intake forms and conduct an initial therapy session.

● Izad Finds Forgiveness

Izad, a single, cisgender man of unknown (by me) sexual orientation, came to the United States from Iran with his family when was 14. He had a psychotic break in his mid-40s when his mother died, an unusual age for a first episode of psychosis. When I asked what brought him to treatment, he replied that his primary care doctor had made the appointment, and we had the following conversation.

THERAPIST: Why did your doctor want you to have therapy? (*Izad looks down and doesn't answer.*) Do you know? (*Izad nods.*) Is it okay to ask? (*He nods, I wait.*)

IZAD: My brother comes to me.

THERAPIST: Hmmm. This form says you're an only child.

IZAD: (*Nods.*) After seven. Before my mother died, my brother Reza came to her. Now he comes to me.

THERAPIST: What does he want?

IZAD: I don't know.

THERAPIST: You haven't asked?

IZAD: I can't change anything

THERAPIST: Does Reza want you to change something?

IZAD: I don't know. (*A few beats.*) I want to change something.

THERAPIST: Can I ask why?

IZAD: I killed him when I was 7.

THERAPIST: Izad, check on something for me. Are all parts of you—all parts inside—ready to talk about this right now? Ask around.

IZAD: Hmm?

THERAPIST: Just ask inside if it's okay for us to talk about this. (*Izad looks down and we are silent for a few seconds, then he nods.*)

IZAD: I'm afraid.

THERAPIST: Can we talk with the part who's afraid? (*Izad nods.*) What does it say?

IZAD: (*After a short silence.*) Does he want me to join him?

THERAPIST: That's the fear? (*Izad nods.*) If I'm understanding you correctly, your brother Reza comes to you now that your mother has died, but he hasn't told you what he wants. (*Izad nods.*) So the fearful part is guessing? (*Izad nods.*) Why would it guess that Reza wants you to join him?

IZAD: Because I think so.

THERAPIST: You have a part who thinks he wants you to join him? Or it thinks that you *should* join him?

IZAD: I should.

THERAPIST: Is it okay to ask why?

IZAD: He would be here except for me. And I would have gone to be with him sooner except for my mother.

THERAPIST: Your mother wanted you to live? (*Izad nods.*) But this part thinks the 7-year-old should die now that his mother is gone? (*Izad nods.*) How do you feel toward the part who thinks the 7-year-old should die?

IZAD: His mother told him to live.

[*He doesn't answer my question.*]

THERAPIST: Do you see him? (*Izad nods.*) And as you see him, how do you feel toward him?

IZAD: I pity him.

THERAPIST: You have a part who pities him?

[*I use parts language.*]

IZAD: He's alone.

THERAPIST: He's lonely? (*Izad nods.*) He lived because his mother said he had to live and now his mother is gone. (*Izad nods.*) Would the part who pities him be willing to step back a little so you can help him? (*Izad nods, and I wait a few beats.*) How do you feel toward him now? (*Izad weeps.*) Are these tears *for* the 7-year-old or *from* him?

IZAD: For him.

THERAPIST: Is this level of feeling okay? (*Izad nods.*) Does the boy see you? (*Izad nods.*) How does he respond?

IZAD: He's surprised. He thought he was invisible.

THERAPIST: Would he like your help? (*Izad nods.*) How do you feel toward him now?

IZAD: I care.

THERAPIST: What needs to happen?

IZAD: He wants to talk to Reza.

THERAPIST: Does he need your help?

IZAD: I will help. (*Closes his eyes for the first time and is absolutely still, tears seep out of his eyes, and it seems like a long time before they open.*) We went to a restaurant at the beach to celebrate his birthday. He was 5. I chased him. He fell off the terrace.

THERAPIST: Oh, Izad! That must have been so shocking. (*Izad nods.*) What's happening with Reza now?

IZAD: He's taking my hand. He wants to play on the beach. (*Leans over, puts his head in his hands, and sobs.*) He doesn't blame me.

THERAPIST: How does that feel? (*He nods.*) Do the boy and Reza see you? (*Izad nods.*) Do they know who you are? (*Izad nods.*) Would they like to come to the present to be with you? (*Izad nods.*) Does the boy have any burdens from that day?

IZAD: Yes.

THERAPIST: Does Reza need him to keep the burdens? (*Izad shakes his head no.*) Does the boy need them? (*Izad shakes his head again.*) Is he ready to let them go? (*Izad nods.*) He could give them to one of the elements, light, earth, air, water, fire . . . or any other way. (*Izad nods.*) Let me know when that's done.

IZAD: (*After a pause.*) They put it in the water.

THERAPIST: How does he feel?

IZAD: Grateful.

THERAPIST: What does he need going forward? He can invite in anything he needs or wants.

IZAD: He needs to stay with Reza and me.

THERAPIST: Okay. (*After a few beats.*) How does that feel? (*Izad nods positively.*) Anything else?

IZAD: They will stay with me.

Izad became suicidal after his mother's death. When questioned, he reported that his dead brother was visiting him. His primary care doctor thought he was psychotic and referred him for a psychiatric evaluation. During the intake evaluation, which became a therapy session, he was able to unblend from his protectors and help the young part who felt responsible for his brother's death. Izad left feeling relieved. The interactions in this session highlight the importance of listening to clients with a completely open mind. It also illustrates the speed with which a client can access their Self, with an emphasis on the word *can* since accessing the Self can also take a long time.

● But What If This?

Readers may wonder what would have happened if Reza had been angry or had blamed Izad. Let's play that out to see how it might have gone. I'll start where Izad has just helped his 7-year-old part ask Reza why he is appearing to Izad.

IZAD: (*Opens his eyes and pauses to wipe tears away.*) He's mad at me.

THERAPIST: What do you say?

IZAD: I used to tease him. I wanted to die after it happened.

THERAPIST: You had a part who said you should die?

IZAD: I was so ashamed.

THERAPIST: Who shamed you?

IZAD: Me.

THERAPIST: You had a critical part who blamed and shamed you? (*Izad nods.*) And how do you feel toward that part, Izad?

IZAD: My mother told me I had to stay alive.

THERAPIST: So that's why you're still here? (*Izad nods.*) And what does the critic say to you now that your mother is gone?

IZAD: Now you can die.

THERAPIST: Would the critic be willing to take a break and let you help these brothers? (*Izad nods.*) What needs to happen?

IZAD: He wants to tell Reza that he's sorry.

THERAPIST: Is that okay with Reza?

IZAD: He says yes. (*A long silence.*) Izad admitted he was jealous. He thought Reza was special.

THERAPIST: How does Reza respond?

IZAD: He likes that Izad is apologizing. He knows Izad didn't mean to hurt him.

THERAPIST: Does Reza still need Izad to feel guilty about the accident? (*Izad shakes his head.*) Would it be okay with Reza if he lets the guilt go? (*Izad nods.*) Does Izad need to hold onto that guilt for any reason? (*Izad nods.*) Why?

IZAD: He hurt his mother.

THERAPIST: Would he like to say something to her now? (*Izad nods.*) Would Reza like to stay for that? (*Izad nods.*) Okay. Let's invite his mother and her higher Self to join the two of them and you.

[*The boy can't accept any measure of pardon without addressing the injury to his mother as well.*]

● What If That?

When I talk about a parent's higher Self, some clients look puzzled, whereas others don't even pause. If they look puzzled, I'll say something like *We all have a higher Self. You didn't have access to this person's higher Self, but we can call on it now because it exists.* I talk more about this in Chapter 7. The scene between Izad's mother and her children could have played out in any number of directions. We never know where a session will go. The mother (from her higher Self) could rapidly forgive him, like this:

IZAD: She's here.

THERAPIST: What needs to happen?

IZAD: He's begging her to forgive him.

THERAPIST: How does she respond?

IZAD: She hugs him. She hugs them both. It's without question.

THERAPIST: How do you feel toward the 7-year-old now?

IZAD: I know he's not a bad boy.

THERAPIST: Let him know that no one is judging him.

Or Reza might speak for Izad with the mother, like this:

IZAD: Izad couldn't look at her, so Reza asked their mother to forgive him.

THERAPIST: How did her higher Self respond?

IZAD: She forgave him, of course.

Throughout the interaction, whatever happens, each person has a higher Self to call on, just as everyone does in individual, couple, and family therapy.

When a Protector Won't Unblend

Although we aim for unblending from the get-go, it can take a while to win cooperation, and we don't want therapy to stall in the meanwhile. When the client can't access their Self, the therapist's Self simply takes the lead and talks directly with the client's parts. In theory, the therapist's Self is always available for this job. If that's true in practice, this strategy is easy. In IFS, a direct conversation between the therapist's Self and a blended part of the client is called *direct access*. The therapist notices that the client's protectors aren't ready to unblend, points it out, and asks the client for permission to speak with their parts. The therapist then speaks about the client in the third person, talking directly with the blended part about other parts of the client while the client's Self listens. In addition to insight or direct access, an IFS therapist can use other methods to engage parts, such as movement, drumming, sand tray, drawing, and so on. I illustrate the differences between insight and direct access below, and I explain more about how to choose between them.

The example of Ava (below) illustrates direct access. Ava was neglected in childhood. Neglected or exploited children yearn for the love of a kind, attentive parent, and their protective parts have various ways of suppressing or distracting from this yearning. One particularly syntonic, powerful distraction involves delicious, wish-fulfilling fantasies of being special and loved. When reality is harsh, these fantasies are all the more important. And, as we see with Ava, when reality and fantasy coincide due to an attentive romantic partner in adult life, an exile can attach like a limpet to stone, even if that partner is intermittently abusive.

The parts who protect an exile like this will say, *Why trade what we provide* (the fantasy) *for an alien unknown* (the Self)? All kinds of unwanted consequences could ensue. They fear losing their jobs and becoming extraneous. And then what for them? The exile could feel hopeful but be disappointed once again, arousing a suicide part. And then what? Each concern must be addressed. For clients who were severely deprived in childhood, the exile's attachment to the fantasy of a loving caretaker, especially when coupled with real experiences of feeling loved, can be an entrenched obstacle to willingness in therapy.

● Ava: A Part Wants Salvatore, Not Self

Ava was a 45-year-old cisgender, bisexual, single European American woman. Her father (now dead) had been a distant family patriarch; her mother was emotionally disturbed and had been, by turns, neglectful and violently rejecting throughout Ava's childhood. A young, intensely yearning part who felt unloved was, it turned out, living in her heart. As it did not protect anyone else, we knew this part was an exile. Ava called it her *electrocuted cat*. The electrocuted cat had an unrelenting attachment to Ava's ex-boyfriend, Salvatore, who had been, by turns, loving and protective, and then harshly critical and rejecting. After years of conflict and distress compounded by growing signals of impatience from friends and family, Ava's most mature managers ended the relationship with Salvatore. Disregarding the new status quo, the electrocuted cat refused to acknowledge love from other sources and undermined new attachments. Understandably, this behavior made other parts angry.

THERAPIST: I was thinking after you left last week that we haven't been able to help the electrocuted cat.

AVA: Yes.

THERAPIST: Can I talk to it directly? (*Ava nods.*) So, I want to talk to the cat. Are you there? (*Ava nods.*) You've said no one understands you. (*Ava nods.*) What would help?

ELECTROCUTED CAT: Nothing. No one can understand.

THERAPIST: Would it help if Ava, the Ava-who's-not-a-part, went with you into your worst experiences?

ANOTHER PART OF AVA: Oh no!

AVA: (*Chuckles.*) That was a popular suggestion. But yes. The cat would love it.

THERAPIST: Okay. But first everyone has to agree. Can I keep talking with the cat? (*Ava nods.*) So, Cat, are you there? (*Ava nods.*) Do you know the Ava-who's-not-a-part?

ELECTROCUTED CAT: She doesn't care about me.

THERAPIST: How do you know?

ELECTROCUTED CAT: I don't want to meet her!

THERAPIST: That's completely up to you. But if other parts were to agree to let her go with you into your experience, would you be willing to meet her?

ELECTROCUTED CAT: Yes.

THERAPIST: Okay. Let's see who objects.

ANOTHER PART OF AVA: What's the point of this?

THERAPIST: To help the electrocuted cat feel better. Other parts, like you, are fed up with her, right? (*Ava nods.*) Would you like her to feel better?

AVA: (*After a moment.*) Okay.

THERAPIST: If anyone wants us to stop at any point, speak up and we will. That way they don't have to interfere, everyone can just be direct. (*Ava nods.*)

ELECTROCUTED CAT: I have a hole. (*Ava points to her chest.*)

THERAPIST: Is the hole what happened to you?

ELECTROCUTED CAT: Yes.

THERAPIST: What do you want Ava to know about the hole?

ELECTROCUTED CAT: It's empty.

THERAPIST: Would you like help with that?

ELECTROCUTED CAT: Yes.

THERAPIST: Would you let Ava help you?

ELECTROCUTED CAT: I want Salvatore.

THERAPIST: What was the best thing about Salvatore?

ELECTROCUTED CAT: He loved me.

THERAPIST: Where do you find his love now?

ELECTROCUTED CAT: In my toes.

THERAPIST: All the way out there?

ELECTROCUTED CAT: Yes.

THERAPIST: Who keeps it out there?

ELECTROCUTED CAT: The parts who hate him.

THERAPIST: If you could bring his love back to the middle, would it fill the hole?

ELECTROCUTED CAT: Yes.

THERAPIST: I have an idea. Can I tell you? (*Ava nods.*) What if other parts
   agreed for Salvatore's love and Ava to join you in the hole?

AVA: She's thinking about that. . . . But she just wants him.

THERAPIST: She wants him or his love?

AVA: Is there a difference?

THERAPIST: Big difference.

ELECTROCUTED CAT: What's the difference?

THERAPIST: His love is in her toes. Even though other parts associate it
   with him, it really belongs to her.

AVA: She sees what you mean.

THERAPIST: You two could bring that love into the hole just to see how it
   feels.

AVA: The other parts would be okay with that, but she doesn't trust me.

THERAPIST: How do you feel toward her?

AVA: I feel a lot of compassion for her. I understand.

THERAPIST: Tell her what you understand and see if she wants to tell you
   more.

AVA: She doesn't want to be alone.

THERAPIST: How do you feel toward her now?

AVA: I love her.

THERAPIST: Does she feel your love?

AVA: Reluctantly.

THERAPIST: That's up to her.

AVA: Okay.

THERAPIST: What does she need from you?

AVA: For now, this attention is okay.

Initially the cat was afraid that meeting Ava's Self would interfere
with her ability to conjure the great comfort of real and imagined love
from Salvatore. Note that as the cat became more willing to talk, the client took over and reported to me on their communications. Although both
insight and direct access are effective, insight helps the client's parts form
a relationship with the client's Self, so therapy goes faster. But if a part
won't unblend, direct access also works well. It frees parts—at least verbal
ones—to talk about the client with the therapist (for some options to help
nonverbal parts, see Chapter 13 on treatment tips). All the while, the client listens and learns about the part's motives and fears. This triangular

communication arrangement generally helps the client access more interest and kindness toward even very challenging parts, like Ava's electrocuted cat. Eventually (not in this session) the cat took Ava into the hole of emptiness, and they stayed there together till the cat felt comforted and decided to bring Salvatore's love back from the toes, all of which proved helpful.

The Capacity to Separate

Sometimes a protector or an exile will say it can't unblend. Although I've run into plenty of protectors who refused to unblend, including a few who never did unblend during my tenure as their therapist, I've found that even stubborn parts are able to unblend (separate from the Self) when they're willing. They can also separate—unblend—from each other internally. In fact, even fanatically controlling protectors routinely unblend to let other parts do mundane maintenance tasks, make lunch, walk the dog, go to school, go to work, and so on. However, their willingness to let others handle maintenance does not imply a willingness to cede leadership to the client's Self. Similarly, if polarized arguing protectors only have eyes for each other, their problem is unwillingness. As a result, I've come to assume that parts who won't separate could do so if they were willing.

So, what motivates protectors to refuse? They always have valid reasons. For one thing, people often begin therapy without any internal agreement among their parts that therapy is a good idea. And there are plenty of other reasons as well. For example, some protectors fear the client will be rejected again. Some believe that they *are* their job and that they will disappear if they stop doing it. Sometimes two protectors are locked in an intense power struggle (called a *polarity* in IFS), so that neither will take notice of the client's Self or any other part. Sometimes a dominant manager insists that it is the one and only part—it is *me*. And, most common of all, sometimes neither managers nor firefighters want the client to be overwhelmed by an exile's emotional pain. The client's Self is poised to help with all this, but its leadership can only begin by popular demand.

If the therapist is thrown off or discouraged by a lack of cooperation, therapy will go more slowly. We gain traction with protectors by noticing them and offering good-natured, calm attention, as illustrated in the session with Ava. They want to know that they won't disappear if they quit their job, and they want to hear that they will always be indispensable members of the inner community. We invite their concerns and coach clients to do some relational mending outside of sessions if possible. But if a part won't give up any corner of consciousness to the Self, the client will need help from someone—a therapist or a trusted counselor—who can offer the needed compassion, confidence, creativity, and persistence to help the part move from wary blending to willing differentiation.

Conclusion

IFS aims for the client to experience life with their Self in the lead. Neither therapist nor client can take the necessary action—what we call unblending—to accomplish this goal; only parts can do that. For this to happen, they must be willing. Sometimes a client's parts unblend in a snap. Occasionally no part of a client's system is willing to unblend. In between those extremes, protective parts gradually test the waters in response to persuasion and patience, separating more for longer periods of time, until they make enough room for the Self to have an influence. Ironically, the more experience they get of the Self, the more willing they are to unblend.

Although a protector's fears of unblending are indexed to the exile's level of wounding, their willingness to unblend depends a great deal on the therapist. Note that everything I've suggested in this chapter involves attitudes and actions that aim to calm our shaming managers, as well as our clients' shaming managers. Our access to the Self is critical. Our negotiating skills and social graces—our curiosity, kindness, egalitarianism, patience, and respect—set the tone for the client's protectors. We invite, include, and learn from them, but they learn from us, too. We guide the client in addressing their parts' concerns. Finally, when the client's Self is witnessing the experiences of an exile, we reassure any protectors who get anxious and interrupt. When it happens, I count myself lucky to be a third-party witness to deep attachment repair.

CHAPTER 3

All the Ways We Say No

This chapter explores how we balance between accepting and refusing, complying and rebelling, yielding and resisting. As Sigmund Freud observed, we all know how to forget, deny, displace, project, repress, rationalize, undo, and so on. Because not accepting reality leads to trouble, mental health treatment is often built around trying to dismantle nonacceptance tactics, a goal many clients share when they come to therapy. Accepting reality is a tenet of psychological health, right? To grieve and move on we must accept what is. People change once they accept. But nonacceptance tactics substitute for the word *no*—and we all need the word *no*—so I've learned to be cautious about promoting acceptance.

I don't want to promote either acceptance or change unless the client's Self and their parts can agree on what needs to happen. So let's consider the wish list of extreme protectors. The proactive, critical team (manager parts) wants to change the supposed flaws and shortcomings of exiled parts. From their perspective, therapy should support this project. In contrast, the reactive, soothing, and distracting team (firefighter parts) wants to silence shaming managers and numb suffering exiles. As far as they're concerned, these imperative goals require action without concern for consequences. This brings us to the dilemma of exiled parts, who can either tolerate being shamed, ignored, or smothered—or they can rebel and overwhelm the client with negative feelings that activate firefighter parts, often including the one who specializes in suicide.

Each category of part has its own perspective on the status quo and what needs to happen, so who are we siding with when we talk with clients about change or acceptance? We don't actually want our clients to embrace any of the preceding options. Exiled parts don't need to change. Manager parts don't need to do all that shaming. Firefighter parts don't need to relieve the sense of shamefulness by killing the client, either quickly or slowly. No person or part needs to die. Nor do clients need to abide endless mental reruns of excruciating moments that can and should be relegated to the past. The pursuit of the wrong kind of acceptance or change turns therapy into a grim project that clients tolerate only with great patience and bravery because they're desperate for help.

So what do I want for my clients? First, I take their parts seriously, and I want them to know it. I aim to be open to all their parts. Then, I want their parts to entertain the idea that meeting the Self could be safe and beneficial. I trust they know that bad things can happen and that people, including caretakers, can be cruel, sadistic, violent, selfish, and annihilating. Just ask a child which stories they love. *Harry Potter? The Golden Compass?* Some gruesome fairy tale? Children can bear bad things happening, but they don't know how to bear the idea that they are bad. When a child accepts global condemnation of their worth, they're doomed to go on and expend a preponderance of their psychic energy justifying and trying to validate their existence. Adults who come to therapy are still doing this—or their parts are doing it.

The benefits of acceptance or rejection always depend on what is being accepted or rejected. If we track this question with our clients carefully, we can avoid the unforced errors that come when our own parts take the lead in therapy. For example, I once suggested that a client might try accepting a relative's frailties rather than trying to protect or fix the relative out of guilt. Although this skills-based intervention sounded reasonable to me, her polite sidestepping signaled my mistake. I checked inside and realized I had a part who wanted to exile her guilt so she would feel better and I would feel competent. But this guilt was central to her parentified experience in childhood. Had she complied and tried to banish her guilty-feeling part, we would have missed an important opportunity to connect with a dominant protector. Change and acceptance of bad luck don't heal; they are the natural outcomes of healing. Until exiles are healed, protective parts will do their job, which may involve trying to change an exile, distract from emotional pain, or parent caretakers. Our goal is not to prevent them from doing these jobs but to remove the necessity.

So Many Ways of Saying No

The word *no* is the North Star of a 2-year-old's life and remains crucial to asserting agency throughout life. But for many children, *no* is a dangerous word. If we can't say *no* directly, our protective parts find alternatives. Freud's *defense mechanisms*, the nonacceptance tactics mentioned earlier, describe some popular options. Before turning to them, let's first consider the differences between defending against something and coping with it. Phebe Cramer (2006) explained that coping strategies are conscious attempts to manage, solve, or change a situation or our reaction to the situation. In contrast, "defense mechanisms occur without conscious effort . . . , operate outside of our awareness . . . , [and] work by changing our internal psychological state—the way we feel, see, or interpret a situation" (p. 20). Following are the salient features of Cramer's defense mechanism theory, translated into parts language.

1. All defenses may have origins in an inborn reflex (such as an infant shutting its eyes if a face looms too close) and the voluntary motor reactions that derive from that reflex (such as moving back if someone gets too close for comfort), which eventually transform into psychic defenses (p. 22). In this way, they appear and are used on a developmental continuum and are connected to the child's cognitive maturity. For example, *denial*, in which an individual fails to "see, recognize, or understand the existence or the meaning of an internal or external stimulus" (p. 23), is available from infancy on but begins to be replaced by around age 7 with the more sophisticated defense of *projection*, in which unacceptable feelings, thoughts, and intentions are attributed to someone else. Projection is, in turn, gradually eclipsed in adolescence by the defense of *identification*, in which the attitudes, beliefs, values, and behaviors of someone else are taken as one's own. "Whereas denial and projection tend to distort reality, identification functions by bringing about a change in the self" (p. 23).
   - In parts language: A child's parts use different protective strategies depending on the child's level of cognitive development.
2. Stress, inside or out, increases the use of defenses.
   - In parts language: When an individual is subject to stressors, inside or out, their protective parts use defenses that suit their own age, temperament, ability, and experience.
3. Defenses should reduce the subjective experience of anxiety.
   - In parts language: Protective parts use defenses to reduce their anxiety about the shamefulness of exiled parts and the behaviors of other protectors.
4. Defenses are effective because they operate outside of awareness, and awareness "should render the defense ineffective" (p. 18).
   - In parts language: Defenses are most effective when other parts and other people view them as somehow inevitable or beyond control. Protectors will say things like *This is just how it is*, or *This can't change*. They prefer to operate behind a curtain, like the Wizard of Oz, and, at least at first, they often express discomfort when they are noticed.

Cramer posits that making the unconscious conscious will render a formerly unexamined defense ineffective, but that is not my experience. Parts can always keep doing what they do. We can't control them, and awareness doesn't prevent them from continuing to use any given defense. However, just as the machinations of the Wizard Oz were cut down to size when his supplicants finally saw him, awareness does seem to deflate the power and influence of a defense. This may be one reason why firefighter parts pinch hit for each other when treatment shines a light on their efforts.

5. "Excessive use of defenses . . . is associated with psychopathology" (p. 18).
   • In parts language: The more active and polarized a person's protectors are, the more likely it is that the person will get a psychiatric diagnosis.
6. While "use of age-inappropriate, immature defenses is associated with psychopathology . . . use of mature defenses is associated with healthy adaptation" (p. 18).
   • In parts language: Young parts don't belong in the driver's seat.

EXERCISE

Identification

Think of someone who influences you in a positive way and consider these questions.

Do you have a part or parts who identify with this person?
What do they value most about this person?
What have your parts learned from this person?

Think of someone who influences you in a negative way and consider these questions.

Do you have a part or parts who identify with this person?
What is most important to that part (or parts) about emulating this person?
What have your parts learned from this person?
Would they like your help to differentiate from this person?

Disowned versus Owned Behaviors

Now let's take a look at how protectors behave. When a person is young and powerless, or for some other reason has little agency to affect the external world, their protective parts will exert influence as they can, which mostly means they will affect their individual's behavior by manipulating perceptions and thoughts. Both Sigmund and Anna Freud described a large number of these tactics (which we've been calling *nonacceptance tactics*), most of which are blunt manipulations of perception or thought that aim to manage anxiety, fear, shamefulness, and anger.*

As Cramer pointed out, early dangers evoke developmentally young tactics. She offers a developmental timeline only for denial, projection, and identification, but readers may want to hazard a guess with the other defenses mentioned below. After years of asking protectors how old they are, I've developed a predictive sense, and I bet you will, too. Following is a list (in alphabetical order) of common defenses, with the Freudian concept first (taken from PsychCentral at *https://psychcentral.com/lib/15-common-defense-mechanisms*), followed by an example, and then my restatement of the defense in parts language.

To Act Out

Freud: To *act out* is to perform an action rather than noticing and tolerating the impulse to perform it without acting.

- For example, a client who has been sober for several months is shamed by their boss and goes directly to a bar after work to drink.

From the IFS perspective, reactive protectors (firefighters) take action to override the inhibitions (shaming) of proactive protectors (managers) in order to distract from the feelings of vulnerable parts who feel shameful (exiles). Note that shaming managers become the intermediary, the internal purveyor, of an insult that was originally external.

To Deny

Freud: To *deny* is to know something but not accept it.

- For example, a man comes to therapy and reports that his childhood was *normal* and *pretty good*. He has a violent temper and becomes suicidal after getting angry. After spending a holiday with his parents, he returns to therapy and reveals that his mother assaulted him physically on more than one occasion during his childhood, always when they were alone. In the next sentence, he denies this, warning the

---

* For a thorough discussion of defense mechanisms, see George E. Vaillant's two books, *Ego Mechanisms of Defense: A Guide for Clinicians and Researchers* (1992) and *The Wisdom of the Ego* (1993). In the latter, Vaillant wrote, "Much of what is labeled mental illness simply reflects our 'unwise' deployment of defense mechanisms. If we use defenses well, we are deemed mentally healthy, conscientious, funny, creative, and altruistic. If we use them badly, the psychiatrist diagnoses us ill, our neighbors label us unpleasant, and society brands us immoral."

therapist not to believe the story. For a few minutes, he goes back and forth between wondering whether it could be true and denying it, as if two different people are speaking. He seems genuinely confused. Did it happen or is he making it up?

From the IFS perspective, protectors who refuse to acknowledge an experience are taking a developmentally young, simple step to handle dangerous information.

To Displace

Freud: To *displace* is to direct an aggressive impulse toward a substitute (less powerful) target.

- For example, a client is shamed by their boss in front of colleagues and then goes home from work and shames their partner or one of their children.

From the IFS perspective, this protector is tossing the hot potato of shamefulness. They are recovering their sense of validity and power after being shamed by causing a vulnerable other to feel small and powerless. However, if a protector shames a therapist (rather than being critical of someone who is truly vulnerable), we can assume the part is engaging the therapist in problem solving. It is posing a question that is very relevant for therapy: *How do you handle being judged and humiliated?*

To Identify with an Aggressor

Freud: To *identify with the aggressor* is to copy an aggressor's behavior after being victimized.

- Protective parts act like an aggressive person from the client's life.

From the IFS perspective, protectors copy an aggressor to exert control over the client (or other people) with the aim of keeping the client safe. For example, the part might believe that shaming will inhibit the client from taking risks that would expose them to more danger or that shaming someone else will make the client feel bigger in comparison to a diminished other.

To Project

Freud: To *project* is to attribute one's own thoughts, feelings, and motives to someone else.

- For example, a teenager clings to their parents and accuses the parents of clinging to them.

From the IFS perspective, protectors keep unacceptable feelings, thoughts, action urges, or behaviors out of awareness by insisting that some other person is feeling, thinking, or acting that way.

To Engage in Projective Identification

Freud: Relatedly, to engage in *projective identification* is not only to insist that someone else is feeling your feelings or has your intentions but also involves taking action to induce those feelings and intentions in the other person.

- For example, accusing someone of vengefulness and then shaming them until they feel vengeful.

From the IFS perspective, a protective part disowns the unacceptable feeling, thought, action urge, or behavior of another part by insisting that someone else feels, thinks, and acts that way and then proves the point by provoking that person to feel, think, or act that way. The term *gaslighting*, which is currently much in vogue, refers to this behavior.

To Rationalize

Freud: To *rationalize* is to make an event or impulse less threatening through cognitive distortion, repression, or ignorance.

- For example, a protector excuses an ethically questionable (but in some way personally profitable) behavior and is completely unconcerned with the consequences for other people. Or a protector excuses the unethical or threatening behavior of someone else in order to avoid confrontation.

From the IFS perspective, protective parts assert a distorted view of our behavior (or someone else's) to benefit us materially, emotionally, or in self-image.

To Repress

Freud: To *repress* is to be unaware of unacceptable thoughts, feelings, and impulses.

- For example, a person has no memory of a frightening event.

From the IFS perspective, protectors keep the thoughts, images, and feelings of traumatically frightened parts (the ones we call exiles) completely out of awareness.

To Undo

Freud: Finally, to *undo* is to make something "un-happen." "Through the use of undoing, individuals try to *symbolically* revert not only the consequences of an event but the event proper, as if it had never existed" (Costa, 2017). If you listen to yourself and others, you will find that undoing is popular.

- For example, a woman who was in a car accident that was fatal for the other driver thinks obsessively about all the things she could do to prevent the accident (which has already happened) from happening (leave 10 minutes earlier, and so on).

From the IFS perspective, an undoing protector goes back to before an event happened to prevent it from happening by imagining behaving differently or imagining getting someone else to behave differently. From the perspective of the material world in which time only goes forward, these efforts are, at best, educational (*I'll never make that mistake again*) and, at worst, absurd (we can't raise the dead). The undoing strategy, which comes easily to parts who hop around in time, succeeds for a moment in postponing an unwanted reality, but, of course, can't undo that reality in the material world. Instead, undoing holds the bad thing in suspended animation, a charged-up, perpetually imminent occurrence that always requires prevention, which makes it a never-ending threat to be feared and avoided rather than grieved. Undoing prevents us from ever completing and coping with the aftermath of events that are, in reality, finished.

Parenthetically, we also seek ways to counter undoing. Consider, for example, that both the jaunty new age aphorism *If it happened it was meant to happen* and the confounding Buddhist statement *You are perfect as you are* may be interrupting undoing protectors rather than aiming for accuracy. Loch Kelly, an IFS-trained Buddhist teacher, takes a tack in the same direction in one of his meditations when he asks listeners to consider, *What's here now when there is no problem to solve?* (see Kelly's [2015] book *Shift into Freedom* or his website).

Apophenia

In addition to all of these protections, we have other common and important ways of acquiring a sense of agency. One is making meaning. When we make meaning to face down chance and bad luck, we are engaging in *apophenia*. Children's parts are particularly good at inventing stories that give them fictional control, and grown-ups who do it are probably blended with young parts. In any case, apophenia comes with the risk of feeling responsible, which is to say guilty, when problems arise. Here's an example. In 1965 a child in New York City was casually hitting light poles with a stick on his way home from school when a huge power blackout hit the East Coast and caused many problems. Upon hearing the news about all these consequences, he was smitten with guilt and stopped speaking. His parents were only able to discover the root of his crisis with much coaxing and the help of a child psychiatrist. I could cite numerous other examples from my therapy practice. One client, for example, confessed that her father had died in a car crash because she was angry with him. Although this belief was an obvious distortion, young parts can also make spurious connections that sound plausible. Rather than arguing, I ask clients if they agree with their parts. If the part remains blended and the client repeats the extreme belief verbatim, then my job is to help the part unblend so the client can access a broader view and reach a more mature verdict on their responsibility.

EXERCISE

An Inquiry with Manager Parts

This exercise gives you an opportunity to hear from one of your managers. You can do this in a number of ways. You might want to read through the instructions and then close your eyes and go through the steps in memory; you might want to record the steps and listen to them; or you might just want to use them for journaling.

Manager parts may get to work very young. When something bad happens, these are the parts who try to figure it out. They're strategic, they're great mimics, and they learn to survive their environment. They take on all the necessary maintenance of life, keep us on track, and care about our relationships with other people. We rely on them. They are the fabric of our social existence. This exercise is intended to help you connect with and appreciate your managers.

Begin by turning your attention inside. You may want to close your eyes, but you don't have to. Do whatever works best for you.

- Invite your managers to join you someplace comfortable and safe, and just see who shows up. As you talk with these parts, make mental notes or pause to journal.
  - Are you there with a part or parts? If you see yourself there, ask the avatar part who's standing in for you to move over and let you be there, too.
  - Do your managers notice you?
    - If not, invite them to notice you.
  - How do they respond?

- o Some may not know who you are or why you called them here. Tell them that you're not here to take anything away.
- o Whatever they want or need, you can help.
- o Ask who wants your attention first.
- o Then ask who that part protects and how.
- o Offer to help the protected part.
- o And then ask the protector what it would rather do if it didn't have to do this job anymore. What does it enjoy?
- Thank it for sharing this information.

The next step is to ask this part (and any other concerned protectors) if it's willing to let you help the exile it just named. If it says yes, set that intention, but don't actually try to help the exile until you've read Chapter 11, in which you will learn how to approach exiled parts safely.

Convincing Protectors to Cooperate

Protectors cooperate when we address their fears. Start by inquiring into motives, which will reveal obstacles to cooperation:

- Ask the part about its motives.
  - o What *would happen if you didn't do this job?*
  - o *Whom do you protect?*
- Listen for:
  - o Loyalty
    - Keep an eye out for parts who use guilt and punishment to tame internal shaming. Their rationale goes something like this: *I'm bad* (my existence hurts others), *but I can atone* (and be good) *by suffering.* This convoluted thinking serves, in their book, to transform badness into goodness.
  - o Responsibility
    - Listen for parts who feel responsible and aim to anticipate or avoid guilt in the future.
  - o Parentification
    - Check for parts who will sacrifice the client to take care of someone else.
  - o Notice dissociative parts.
  - o Does the client space out in the middle of a discussion or in response to a question? Ask what just happened.

- ○ Ask if the client ever experiences a mental vacuum.

  [It's probably a way of keeping exiled parts out of mind.]

  - ▪ If yes, ask to talk with that part directly so the client can listen.
    - □ If the part talks, ask who it protects and what would happen if it stopped.
    - □ If it doesn't speak, it's either not yet willing or it's preverbal.
  - ▪ If it's not yet willing to be in connection, give it a pep talk along these lines: *I know how important you are to Max [the client]. I bet you've been doing this since he was little. And I bet—and I hope you'll correct me if I'm wrong—that you kept him safe in some tricky situations. I think you did a great job because, look, here he is! But you wouldn't have to worry so much or work so hard now if you let the Max-who's-not-a-part help out. Would you like to meet him? He's all about helping you and the parts you protect.*
  - ▪ Preverbal dissociative parts
    - □ Ask the client to notice how the part responds to this patter. They may notice some relaxing, some relief, or some sudden clarity.
    - □ If the part has responded positively, have the client ask what it needs now, and also guide the client in offering to help the part it protects.

● Jo Undoing

The following example illustrates the protection that Freud called undoing. Jo, a 25-year-old, cisgender, single, French-Scottish American person who used the pronoun *they*, grew up in a dangerous, chaotic household with five physically imposing, athletic older siblings. Jo's older brothers got into fistfights with each other and picked fights at school. Their parents were, by turns, neglectful (traveling often and leaving Jo in the care of their eldest sister, who could be violent), intrusive (when Jo was 5 years old their mother removed all the doors in the house), volatile, and passionately engaged with each other. Jo was the last to leave home for college but came and went from college a few times (the impetus for therapy) before finishing and getting a job. Within a few months they got fired from the job after arguing with their boss. A week later, they arrived in therapy with a cardboard shoebox in hand and placed it on the floor between us.

Jo: My bird Chirper. (*Takes the lid off the box to reveal a dead parakeet.*)
THERAPIST: Chirper died. (*Jo nods silently.*) Who needs attention?

Jo: I went out and forgot to leave the light on. He got cold. I should have left the light on and put the blanket over the cage to keep him warm.

Therapist: You have a part who says you could have kept him alive?

Jo: He was old.

[*This is another part.*]

Therapist: One part tells you that you could have kept him alive, and another reminds you that he was old?

Jo: I've been keeping him in the freezer.

Therapist: Because?

Jo: I was going to bury him, but I had a dream that he was alive and a cold draft was blowing through the house. When I woke up, I couldn't decide if he was dead or alive, so I put him in the freezer.

Therapist: You have a part who wants to prevent his death? (*Jo nods.*) What is it concerned would happen if it stopped trying to do that?

[*This part is undoing Jo's current reality. If I didn't know Jo, I would think they were psychotic.*]

Jo: He would die.

Therapist: The part doesn't know that he is dead?

Jo: It doesn't want me to think about that.

Therapist: What is it concerned would happen if you thought about Chirper's death?

Jo: I'd feel too sad.

[*This is the exile.*]

Therapist: If you could help the one who feels sad, would this part still need to stop Chirper from dying?

[*Pairing the problem behavior (undoing) with the part's protective intent.*]

Jo: Not really.

Therapist: Would it let you help the sad part? (*Jo nods.*) Does anyone else object?

Jo: Yes. Other parts are afraid of the sadness.

Therapist: What scares them most?

Jo: I'll get overwhelmed and . . . die.

Therapist: A suicide part would step in? (*Jo nods.*) And who do these worried parts think you are?

Jo: (*After a pause.*) A kid.

Therapist: How old is the kid?

Jo: Seven.

[*I assume this 7-year-old is the exile, though I could be wrong.*]

THERAPIST: Can the scared parts see you as well as the 7-year-old?

JO: Yes.

THERAPIST: Will you be overwhelmed by the 7-year-old, Jo?

JO: No.

[*Jo has enough Self-energy now to feel confident that negative feelings won't be overwhelming. This is new.*]

THERAPIST: But some other parts are afraid of being overwhelmed by the 7-year-old's sadness. Let them know you can handle this.

[*When managers say they're afraid of emotional overwhelm, they mean they fear being overwhelmed—as in, knocked out of the spotlight by the panicked, dangerous reactivity of firefighters. The Self may be pushed out of awareness, but it's not overwhelmed by feelings.*]

JO: They don't trust me.

THERAPIST: If the 7-year-old is willing to be with you without taking over, you can handle this and everyone else can go to a waiting room.

JO: They want a room with a door.

THERAPIST: Of course. The waiting room will have a door.

This session illustrates an undoing part in action. Its irrationality reminds me that we're talking with a developmentally young part whose imaginative solution to current threats is congruent for the part but can't possibly work in the material world. If I have the urge to argue when a part sounds irrational, I hope to catch my argumentative part before it speaks. My linear thinking doesn't help undoing protectors feel better connected or safer. My aim, as illustrated in the preceding dialogue, is to stay curious and find out who this part protects.

The Magicians of the Psyche at Work

Protectors exert influence where they can. In the process, they make ample use of the variations on *no* listed earlier. Managers are too rule-bound to pass for rebels, but their efforts are geared to resisting the ruinous fate of unlovability, which they do to the best of their ability. The true rebels—reactive firefighter parts who aim for relief from current managerial shaming, the exiled feeling of shamefulness, and external insults—are also managing the problem of feeling unlovable. As they escape emotional pain by not knowing, distracting, refusing, being someone else, getting someone else to be me, manipulating time, and so on, their overall message—*Look! I am a magician*—is so true in the psyche but so false in the material world.

Rather than arguing with their tactics, we ask (rhetorically, as we know the answer), *Is it effective?* And then we offer something new.

In general, the more we respect and admire refusal, repudiation, denial, negation, and noncompliance, the better we do with protectors. After all, how can anyone survive without having the will and ability to say no? Although protective tactics create many secondary problems, we take aim at the underlying, primary problem of emotional pain that goes with feeling unlovable. When no one else was there to help, these protectors showed up and got creative. If we validate their positive intentions and address their fears, they're usually willing to try something new.

Transference Tests

On the rare occasions when a part is unyieldingly resistant, I start thinking in terms of transference, a relational phenomenon in which the client recreates traumatizing interactions from the past in the therapeutic relationship today. Specifically, I think in terms of *transference tests*, a concept Joseph Weiss (1993), a psychiatrist from San Francisco, developed after recording and studying transcripts of his analytic sessions to track how patients (as he called them) made progress in therapy. As Weiss examined his sessions, he concluded that patients use relational reenactments to coach therapists about their needs, and he developed a therapy called Control Mastery, with the word *control* signifying that patients have an unconscious plan for therapy and the word *mastery* signifying their wish to master challenges.

According to Weiss, people arrive in therapy with preformed *pathogenic beliefs*, which largely revolve around survivor and separation guilt. They use therapy to pose what he called *behavioral enactments*, or transference tests, that give the therapist a chance to challenge and disconfirm their guilt-based pathogenic beliefs. Clients heal, according to Control Mastery theory, when therapists pass their tests. In the same vein, though with an emphasis on shame rather than guilt, IFS sees the client's Self challenging the shaming beliefs of exiled parts and sees clients healing when their exiled parts release these burdensome beliefs. I find the IFS approach is effective with both shame and guilt as long as protectors cooperate. But if we can't get traction with them and reach the client's Self, Weiss's idea of transference tests can come in handy. Here is an example. A miscommunication about an appointment time gave one of my clients the opportunity to reenact a problem that they had not been able to reveal directly. I believe this client's protectors needed to know that I could be trusted in deeds as well as words. Their opportunity to find out unfolded in this way.

Believing that my next hour was unscheduled, I mistakenly left the client sitting in the waiting room for 20 minutes. Once I realized my mistake, I apologized and gave her a choice. We could reschedule the session or go ahead and meet at a prorated fee. The client calmly opted for the shorter session but said she would still pay the full fee. Finding her affect and her offer puzzling, I reiterated that I would cut the fee for a curtailed session. In the remaining time (about 35 minutes), she disclosed for the first time that her mother had trained her to shoplift when she was 8 years old. From the Control Mastery perspective, I had passed a transference test, and she, in turn, had revealed a tender secret about being criminally exploited by her mother.

This example illustrates a client recreating a traumatic power dynamic in therapy by casting herself in the more vulnerable role, just as she had been in childhood, and casting me in the powerful role of potential exploiter. It was a direct reenactment of her childhood. When I declined to exploit her, she felt safer and revealed a secret. Weiss called this a *direct* transference test, but the reverse—when the client takes the more powerful position and gives the therapist the less powerful role of the child—he called a *passive-into-active* transference test. The latter is more challenging for the therapist, and clients will only do it when they trust the therapist to handle the test skillfully, without collapsing or attacking.

Another client of mine, Bjorn, provides an example of a passive-into-active transference test. Bjorn was shaken up when his former lover refused to repay a large loan and accused him of being heartless and greedy for asking. Because she was keeping his money without apparent remorse, this is a good example of projection—she was projecting her heartless greed onto him. Soon after their interaction, Bjorn started missing therapy appointments without giving an excuse or notifying me. When I billed him for the sessions, he got angry. We could say that his protector was using the Freudian defense of identification with the aggressor and casting me in the vulnerable role of receiving that aggression, which was Bjorn's actual experience with his ex-girlfriend.

Predictably, a couple of my parts took umbrage at his behavior, feeling demeaned and annoyed. But I explained that his behavior was an invitation to pass a therapeutic test and they calmed down. Then I did two things. First, I didn't budge on billing him for the missed sessions. Second, I asked him, with genuine curiosity, to check inside and find out what was going on. In response, he escalated and accused me of being greedy and not caring about him. If my protectors had counterattacked (*It's in our agreement, I'm being perfectly reasonable, let's take a look at your behavior*) or if I had been compliant (*I'm so sorry! I don't want to jeopardize our connection, money isn't important*), I would have failed the test, Bjorn would have felt less safe, his therapy would have stalled, and he would have been less likely to assert himself in other relationships. I passed the test by being firm as well as curious. Bjorn stopped missing sessions and started talking about his childhood relationship with his father, a bitingly critical man. He spoke of asking his father to stop shaming him with mean jokes. In response, his father had accused Bjorn of being the shamer. Bjorn didn't know how to respond to this reversal. When he recreated the same dynamic with me years later, my response modeled an adaptive way of handling humiliating aggression.

If we can coax protectors to unblend, we do not have to establish relational safety through risky, energy-draining reenactments of attachment trauma. When protectors are able to talk about their fears, they don't need to pose transference tests in therapy. But when they do reenact traumatic relational dynamics with us, they need an appropriate response. They want to see someone handle the interaction with courage, confidence, and compassion rather than helplessness, self-blame, or rage. They want to let go of the pathogenic beliefs we're calling burdens. The Control Mastery approach is thus very compatible with IFS. It is useful if a client reenacts a trauma rather than hearing about it from their parts. When I feel I'm being recruited to play a role from the client's past, I assume that past is still, for whatever reason, unspeakable. By passing their transference test, I toss a lifeline to a part who is muted and stuck in a scary place back then.

Conclusion

To navigate relationships, we need a genuine *yes* and a genuine *no*. Especially, we need a genuine *no* to shaming. Because many clients grow up in circumstances in which *yes* and *no* are not options, their protective parts take evasive action. We've looked at how Sigmund and Anna Freud viewed those evasions, and I've given examples of three Freudian defenses that can be particularly confusing: undoing, projecting, and identifying with an aggressor. I've also described how I focus on passing transference tests when a protector acts instead of unblending. I'll end this chapter by saying that the evasive actions of blended protectors work in the short run but cost too much over time. However, they won't stop until the Self is available to help with *yes* and *no*.

CHAPTER 4

The Shame Cycle

When exiles show the Self how they developed such negative beliefs about who they are, they generally return to shaming (sometimes terrifying) interactions that preceded the client's feeling shameful and precipitated what I call the *shame cycle*, which is the topic of this chapter. The shame cycle starts with an event. Perhaps an adult or an older child assaults a child physically or sexually. Or someone (or an event) shames the child for a behavior (*you're too loud, too quiet, too slow, too fast . . .*), or a need (*you're too demanding, too hungry, too close, too distant . . .*), or an attribute of their body (*your feet are too big, your nose isn't right, you're too short, too tall, too large, too small . . .*). The child may also be dissatisfied because their body isn't functioning well or can't perform as they wish.

If a quality of the psyche draws shaming, we'll call it a part; if the object of shaming is an attribute of the body, we'll consider how parts feel toward the body as a result. In both cases, shaming extrapolates from the particular to the whole, from the attribute (too much or not enough of something) to identity (*you are . . . worthless, unlovable, bad, defective*). As a result, parts receive targeted criticisms as global condemnations. In response, protectors want to *do* something. But what can they do?

Listen for conjugations of the verb *do* in therapy and you'll locate the client's activist shame protectors: *What can I do? I don't know what to do! I did this for them. If I stop doing this, what else will I do?* Should they defend the injured part at the expense of the whole, or defend the whole and sacrifice the part? Generally, they sacrifice the part. If someone tells me I'm too loud, my managers tell me to be quiet; if someone tells me I'm too tall, they tell me to slump; if I struggle with math lessons and get criticized

54

or someone tells me I'm not capable of learning math, they draw a curtain over numbers; and so on. Of course, sometimes the protective response is to approach and overcome obstacles rather than hiding and avoiding. For example, I'm dyslexic, so I become a writer; I have a speech impediment, so I become a politician; I had to wear a back brace as a child, so I become a dancer. Although the latter responses are more likely to feel (and be) productive, if a shamed part has been exiled and papered over in the process of overcoming obstacles, then the same internal dynamic still applies, and the same kind of suffering is going on somewhere in the nether reaches of the psyche.

When a child is shamed by more powerful others, sacrificing the part for the whole is a sensible move. Our social guardians, proactive managers, won't allow the whole system to be judged for some attribute of the body or a single psychic part. They aim to fix or eliminate the offending part, they're willing to work at becoming acceptable, and their opening gambit usually involves a lot of shaming. Once inner shaming begins, ironies abound. The child who was shamed is no longer just a recipient of shaming, they are now also the shamer. And their shaming, which becomes a chronic bloodletting over time, spawns a whole new set of problems.

Six Acts

At the outset of therapy, the initial shaming event—and the child's acceptance of that shaming as valid information—is history. The client may not disclose that history or even recognize its relevance, but the therapist will certainly hear how their protectors have been handling it. To make this clear, I divide the following story into six distinct acts in the way a play is typically divided into two or three acts. The first act is the prompting event, the second act is the individual's response to that event. After this come four more acts in which protective parts take steps to handle the prompting event and its acceptance in the first two acts. I present all this in a certain order, but, in reality, only the prompting event and the individual's initial acceptance of shaming have a necessary chronology. The daisy chain of protective responses that occurred thereafter and continue in the present can come in any order. Additionally, once these responses get going, more than one can be happening at the same time, because more than one part can be active at a time. Ultimately, as I illustrate, their order is less important than how they reinforce each other.

In the first act, the prompting event occurs. A child is shamed (act 1). In the second act, the child accepts that shaming as valid information about who they are (act 2). In the third act, a team of proactive internal managers mobilizes to shame the part who was shamed (act 3). Clients give these parts names—such as the *critic, judge, censor, expert, monitor, analyst, evaluator*—or they experience the actual external critic as being inside their psyche, and so on. In the fourth act, another team of managers comes online to anticipate and prevent future external shaming by repeatedly warning the client not to behave in ways that will evoke shaming (act 4). These parts are fearful scouts who get out in front to anticipate danger. In the fifth act, a team of reactive warrior parts (i.e., firefighters) activate to shame other people (act 5). Their goal is to distract from inner shaming and toss the hot potato of shamefulness to someone else. Finally, in the sixth act, another team of reactive protectors (also firefighters) steps in with disinhibited behaviors, including addictive processes such as drinking, drugging, porn use, risky sexual encounters, video gaming, binge-watching TV, raging, extreme uses of food, and so on (act 6). These parts ignore long-term consequences in favor of immediate physical and psychic relief.

When therapy begins, the dominant team earns the client a diagnostic label and provides the rationale for treatment. High-risk clients often earn a long list of diagnoses as they move through treatment systems, with reactive protectors pushing back in various ways against critics, inside and out, on a daily or even hourly basis. We find polarized protectors competing for control in order to ward off a suicide part. For example, a manager says to get sober, whereas a firefighter says have a drink; or reactive protectors have control and pinch hit for each other. For example, when a drinking part steps back, an eating disorder part steps in.

In general, protective parts aim to put historical injuries out of mind or minimize them, and when the parts who were injured do get into consciousness (even with permission), the enormity of their experience can still overwhelm other parts. On the other hand, some historical events look far less significant from an adult perspective and relative to the havoc protectors wreaked thereafter. In this case, a client may find it hard to credit the exile's revelations as relevant, and protectors may argue that something truly terrible must still be repressed. We should not make the mistake of assuming this is true. Once we've helped the client track through the various attempted solutions to manage the exile's injury, introduced the Self, and helped protectors calm down, it's crucial to validate the significance of whatever the exile discloses.

Hugh's experience is a good example. He felt he couldn't progress in life. He was drinking too much and wasn't finishing the research required to get his PhD in physics. When he went inside during therapy sessions, he saw swirling colors and couldn't make contact with any particular part. Fast forward 18 months. Hugh was in a session and asked all his protectors to gather round and talk with him. A group of tall, ghostly figures appeared. One of them sat at the far end of their big council table holding a 3-year-old boy on its lap. Meanwhile, another reminded him of a story. When Hugh was 3 years old he begged his uncle to pick him up. His uncle laughed, bent down, and then collapsed on the floor in a cry of pain. A disc had fractured, and he was taken by ambulance to the hospital, where he underwent surgery. He was never as physically robust again, and Hugh's parts had always believed the 3-year-old was responsible. More broadly, they still believed that Hugh's needs were dangerous, bad, and shameful.

At the end of that session, Hugh looked at me in astonishment and said, "*That* was it?" He could not believe it. Everyone in Hugh's family understood that his uncle's back had been damaged prior to this collapse, no one had ever blamed Hugh, and everyone had always been kind and supportive. His current angst puzzled them as much as him. Yet the ghostly figures, protectors of the little boy, had come when he called and stared at him with baleful eyes, clutching the little boy away from him—and from the team of critical managers who blamed the boy and were generally blended with Hugh. Yes, indeed. That was it.

One caveat about internal critics. They are different from external critics. Although they may sound and look like an external critic, they intend good things for the recipient of their shaming. Rather than perpetuating the bad thing that happened, they aim to prevent it from happening again. Although their behavior reinjures the shamed part, they mean to make the part worthy of love. They are usually young and don't see the irony of criticizing someone to prevent them from being criticized, and they don't remotely understand how internal shaming transforms a painful external interaction into a dangerous identity that revolves around a sense of worthlessness. Trapped in a single-minded, developmentally young dedication to shaming, they don't actually want to be reinforcing the substrate of loneliness, despair, and desolation they help to create.

In act 4, some vigilant, anticipatory scout parts go to work. These parts are allergic to feeling powerless, weak, scared, and excluded. They fear the future. They live on high alert and look for danger down the road. They try to scare us into doing this and not being that. They focus on social etiquette, and they prioritize meeting the needs and demands of other people. To preempt disaster, they imagine, revisit, and rehearse. They dredge up scenes of embarrassment from the past and show us how we might be shamed in the future. They tell us what to care about, who to be, and how to fit in. From the clothes we wear to the language we use, from the ideas we entertain to the people we pursue, anticipatory shamers take pains to help us belong. They warn us to stick with the group. Their dread of being shamed cues us up to the dangers of being different and the looming peril of exile. It pushes us to comply with group norms. Think, for example, of how important wardrobe choices are for adolescents.

Conformism is a prosocial but not necessarily beneficial behavior. People who participate in lynch mobs are conforming to a group. The longing to belong in groups can eclipse concern and compassion, leading protective parts to transgress. No one in a lynch mob is exercising critical judgment about the beliefs and behavior of the group. And no one is immune from the comfort of seeing through the eyes of a group that keeps them safe from accountability. Anticipatory protector parts drive us toward conformism. They want us to please others and be popular externally. But because they manufacture anxiety, they are not popular internally. As we consider their role, we need to distinguish between the negative effects of their behavior, when these occur, and their prosocial intent. Their desire to avoid more shaming is a reasonable but, for practical purposes, impossible goal that leaves us more, not less, vulnerable to being shamed and to the antisocial reactivity of protective parts in acts 5 (shaming others) and 6 (self-soothing and distracting without concern for costs).

When we reach the last two acts of the shame cycle, the Spartan self-sacrifice, fearful warnings, and chronic self-neglect that inner critics promote comes home to roost and inspires the opposite. Acts 5 and 6 can come in any order or occur in close conjunction, but I discuss act 5 (shaming others) first. We all shame. Our protectors might shame in subtle, disowned ways (what we now call a *microaggression*) or in purposeful, blatant ways that are out in the open. In either case, act 5 protectors turn festering insults outward. They seek to hand despised qualities off to someone else—*you, not me.* These disowned qualities need not be true of the other person because the point of shaming is to bring at least temporary relief to the internal system of the shamer with the assurance *I am not that.*

Finally, in act 6, soothing and distracting firefighters activate with shameless, quick-fix indulgences (or the opposite, extreme restraint) that range from eating disorders and addictive processes to rage and suicide. The intent of disinhibited protectors is prosocial in the sense that they're concerned about the well-being of the internal system. But because they're not concerned about the fears of manager parts, consequences to the body, or the needs and comfort of other people, their behavior is antisocial in effect. If firefighter parts register other people, they are a means to an end. This lack of concern makes them shameproof. They want relief from pain in the body and mind right now. They can never achieve lasting relief, but, equally, the manager parts of other family members and treaters can't shame them into quitting. On the contrary, because external shaming inflames exiled pain, it hardens their resolve to keep on helping. When we shame ourselves, we make a bad experience into a painfully false identity, which, in turn, generates bad behavior. When we shame others, we spread unease, pollute our relational environment, and grant the shame cycle a plaguing immortality.

So that's how the shame cycle goes. Someone, usually an adult, an older child, a peer, or an event—but sometimes just a proactive part of the child who notices that the child is different—shames the child. That shaming may present in the guise of caretaking, or it may be direct and purposeful. Violence and sexual behavior that adults (or older kids) direct at children are shaming. Neglect and disregard are shaming. Invalidation is shaming (*No, you don't want that candy*). Any behavior that says *I don't see you; you don't matter* or *I will use you* is shaming. Because dependency primes us to accept external judgments, children are exceptionally vulnerable. A child who has enough external support (and is able to admit they need it) can get help to challenge outside judgments and avoid taking on the burden of shamefulness. But the child who accepts shaming is trapped in the cycle I've described. Whether shame is explicitly named or not during the course of therapy, we explore this cycle in therapy. Acts 1 and 2 often go unmentioned as the client begins therapy. They are the hidden history of exiled parts. In contrast, acts 3 through 6 are already in motion. Here we find the critics, anticipatory scouts, warriors, and distractor/soothers doing their thing.

The Shame Cycle in 6 Acts

Act 1. Injury: A Bad Thing Happens

- An authority figure (caretaker, relative, teacher, older child, sibling, or peer) shames a child.

The shamer is *not me*. This bad thing that happens is interpersonal. The shamed child is a passive recipient of the shaming with no intent in this situation. Flash forward to therapy in the present. Now the bad thing that happened is history.

Act 2. Acceptance: The Shamed Part Believes *I Am Bad (Defective, Worthless, Evil, Rotten, Monstrous, Too Much, Too Little)*

- The shamed part accepts the judgment and concludes *I am shameful.*

Acceptance, like the event itself, predates and sets the stage for the problems the client brings to therapy.

Act 3. Critics Go Large: *That's True, You Are Bad*

- Some proactive manager parts hold the shamed part of the child responsible for being shamed, and they shame it, hoping it will improve or at least lie low.

I call this *instrumental shaming* because, even though it will eventually lead to antisocial avoidance and reactive rage, this inner shamer has a positive, prosocial intent. It aims to take control in a dangerous situation. It inhibits the shamed part, who it views as a liability, in order to stay safe. With the advent of inner shaming, *I* become the shamer as well as the recipient of shaming.

Act 4. Prevention: Never Again

- Anticipatory scout managers take on the job of warning the individual. They aim to prevent more shaming, inside or out, by anticipating the complaints of a (real or imagined) critical audience, and they, too, want to improve the shameful part.

The scout part who anticipates future shaming maintains a dual focus, at once keeping an eye on internal vulnerability and external dangers. Unlike the exiled part who passively receives shaming, scout parts are active. They aim to take control; they believe in surviving by belonging. Because of them and other critical parts, a problem that was once external becomes self-generated. Their intent is prosocial, but their actions reinforce the antisocial existence of exiled parts and the antisocial behavior of firefighter parts.

Act 5. The Warrior Mutiny: *No, You Are Bad*

- Some reactive firefighter parts shame other people, diminishing them by comparison and rebooting the self-esteem of a system that is collapsing under the weight of internal shaming.

I call this *external instrumental shaming.* The reactive part who shames others is externally focused, active, rebellious, and disinhibited. Though its behavior is antisocial and its effect is bound to be antisocial, its internal intent is prosocial. It aims to help a system of parts that is struggling with the assault of continual shaming.

Act 6. The Rescue Team: *Feel Better*

- Meanwhile, other reactive firefighter parts use some preferred way of numbing and/or distracting to get relief from shaming and shamefulness.

A wide range of behaviors involving disinhibition fit the bill for self-soothing or distracting from internal shaming. The firefighters who engage in these behaviors are internally focused, rebellious, and active. They drink too much, use drugs excessively, smoke cigarettes, gobble soothing foods, and generally take risks without concern for what we might call side effects or unintended outcomes. They mean to be helpful inside, and they are asocial interpersonally—they don't care about others—but the effects of their behavior tend to be antisocial and negative.

> **Recovery: *A Bad Thing Happened to Me***
>
> I've organized this cycle neatly into separate acts, but therapy sessions are unlikely to seem neat. After protectors launch, parts in these roles can all be in action simultaneously. As a result, listening to the client's experience can be confusing for the therapist, and experiencing it can be overwhelmingly confusing for the client. Nonetheless, client and therapist can use this framework to locate the different perspectives and agendas of parts who are involved in the shame cycle.

Can Shaming and Shamefulness Be Beneficial?

I would be remiss if I didn't mention that the field of mental health does not agree about the function or usefulness of shame. Many emotion researchers and clinicians have delved into shame, and a great deal has been written on the topic. Alan Schore (1994) pointed out that shaming inhibits young children, which often keeps them from harm. Nonetheless, shaming is a disrespectful behavior that hurts the recipient. Although the caretaker's intent may be protective, it is irrelevant to the child's experience. Despite the (often spectacular) ways in which shaming promotes emotional reactivity and, eventually, disinhibition, it's easy to find proponents of shaming, especially if the shamer is shaming disinhibition (Sykes, 2016; Sykes & Sweezy, 2023). Does the shamer intend to edify? Constrain dangerous, disinhibited behavior? Then, the reasoning goes, shaming is good. Does the shamer intend to intimidate, dominate, exploit? Then shaming is bad. This view focuses on the shamer's intent, not the effects of their behavior. It is magical thinking to assume that my intent will govern your experience.

Even though the effects of shaming are not dependent on the shamer's intentions, it can be tricky to see the difference between intent and outcome. I suspect this is because parts' intentions do matter—but only for one person. My parts' intentions are crucially important to me, but not to you or anyone else. To care for myself responsibly and be considerate of others, I need to understand my parts' intentions, which are always positive for me in some way. But positive intentions for me are simply not relevant for you. First, if my parts are protecting me, they're not thinking about you; and, second, good intent can lead to bad (wounding or transgressive) behavior. Only my behavior matters to you. Shaming isn't educational, it's not a kindness in disguise, it isn't protective, and it's not for your benefit. What do you feel when shamed? You feel hurt.

Our manager parts are likely to count injured feelings as evidence that the insult is accurate. If I feel ashamed, I must be shameful. To avoid that seeming reality, my managers may assign good intentions to the shamer, engage in self-improvement efforts (self-shaming), sign on for shaming as a valid approach to influencing others, and so on. Because their intentions are good, they trust the outcome will be good. Their sincere efforts activate firefighter parts and set the client seesawing between recoil (inhibition and self-attack) and rage (disinhibition), seen in antisocial behaviors, such as shaming others, and in various self-soothing behaviors (that are also antisocial in the long run), such as overusing alcohol, drugs, pornography, and so on. But failure and disappointment just make managers try harder. Authority figures who use shaming to exert influence are playing with fire.

How the Shame Cycle Shows Up in Treatment

Most clients begin therapy somewhere in the middle of their shame cycle, often with many parts being active in various roles at the same time. For example, new clients may shame themselves or someone else as soon as they start either individual or couple therapy (for more on shaming in couple therapy, see Herbine-Blank & Sweezy, 2021). That's the critical team, act 3, at work. Or they may express anxiety about being shamed. That's act 4, the anticipatory warning team. Alternatively, they might shame the therapist or complain about someone else. That's act 5, the warrior team. Or the client might describe being in the grip of compulsive self-soothing. That's the feel-better team of act 6. Whatever one we hear about first, we will eventually hear about some or all of the acts between 3 and 6 as they occur in the client's life today. Here is an example of how I might unpack the shame cycle with one client over time, starting at the beginning of treatment.

Darika was a 26-year-old, cisgender, heterosexual, partnered, first-generation American. Her parents had immigrated to the United States from Delhi, India, before Darika and her two brothers, one older and one younger, were born. Both were professors (her mother of chemistry, her father of medicine) at American universities in two different states, which meant they commuted back and forth. As a result, Darika and her brothers were raised by their maternal grandparents. They attended overwhelmingly European American private schools, and, in ninth grade, Darika went off to a boarding school. Now in her 20s, she had a Ukrainian American boyfriend named Yuri, who was a pleasant fellow unless he was drinking, in which case he was often rude and unpleasant.

● An Example of Act 3: Inner Critics

On the phone before we met, Darika told me that she was in graduate school studying sociology but was on the verge of dropping out. Her older brother was already in residency in medical school and on his way to becoming a surgeon. She said her parents were disappointed that she had decided not to go into science or medicine, and she was having a hard time concentrating in school. Her boyfriend, Yuri, who was trying to launch a career as a freelance journalist, had recently gone off the wagon and was drinking. He had recently moved in with Darika because he was financially strapped. Her family disapproved and wouldn't visit as long as he was living there. Even though she wanted to kick him out, she didn't. So a friend urged her to try therapy. She let me know right away that she was anxious (fearful about the future) and depressed (ashamed regarding the past).

THERAPIST: Which of those needs your attention?

DARIKA: I decide? I thought you'd know.

THERAPIST: Ask inside.

DARIKA: (*After a few beats.*) I guess the anxiety.

THERAPIST: Where do you notice it?

DARIKA: In my stomach.

THERAPIST: How do you feel toward it?

DARIKA: Overwhelmed. My doctor wants to me to take Klonopin, but I'm not going down that road.

THERAPIST: What is the anxiety in your stomach like?

DARIKA: Gnawing?

THERAPIST: How do you feel toward it?

DARIKA: Scared.

THERAPIST: Can you see it?

DARIKA: It's a trapped gerbil.

THERAPIST: It's scared or you're scared of it?

DARIKA: It's scared.

THERAPIST: How do you feel toward it?

DARIKA: I feel sorry for it.

THERAPIST: What scares it?

DARIKA: The meanness.

THERAPIST: Who is mean?

DARIKA: Hmm. Me, I guess.

THERAPIST: You have a mean part? (*Darika nods.*) Would the gerbil feel better if you helped the mean part? (*Darika nods.*) Does anyone else inside object? (*Darika shakes her head.*) Would the gerbil like to go somewhere else while you do that? Somewhere safe. (*Darika nods.*) The gerbil can show you the right place. (*She nods.*) Okay to check in with the mean part now? (*Darika nods.*) Where do you find it?

[The gerbil is Darika's exile; the mean part, who is a protector, needs attention before the exile.]

DARIKA: In my head.

THERAPIST: How do you feel toward it?

DARIKA: It's evil. (*Shrugs.*)

THERAPIST: Ask if it belongs to you.

DARIKA: Yes.

THERAPIST: It's a part of you?

DARIKA: Yes.

THERAPIST: Okay. Ask all the parts who fear or hate it to give you some space. They can go to a waiting room so you can talk with it. (*Darika nods.*) How do you feel toward it now?

DARIKA: I wonder why it does this.

THERAPIST: What does it say?

DARIKA: *You are such a monster. You hate Yuri, but you keep him around. You disappoint your parents. You're a loser.*

THERAPIST: That's what it says when it's doing its job. Is it willing to take a break and talk about why this job is important?

DARIKA: Okay.

THERAPIST: What would happen if it stopped being mean?

DARIKA: I'd get hurt.

THERAPIST: It protects you.

DARIKA: It thinks so.

THERAPIST: What does it want for you?

DARIKA: (*Listens inside.*) It wants me to be loved.

THERAPIST: It wants people to love you. (*Darika nods.*) How do you feel toward it now?

DARIKA: (*Shakes her head.*) I'm surprised.

Thus, Darika met a shaming critic and learned about its intention for her in her first session of therapy. The critic was causing another part of her, a trapped gerbil part, to feel scared and miserable. Its misery and feeling of being unloved was gnawing at her gut. The gerbil wanted Yuri to fix this feeling and couldn't bear the idea of being alone. Under its influence, Darika let Yuri stay in her apartment even though he was drinking and not contributing financially. This enraged the angry critic, who she was calling *mean*.

⬤ An Example of Act 4: The Anticipation Team

Because we're all capable of feeling shameful, we all have parts who anticipate feeling shameful. Their anxiety-producing activity can have advan-
tages. The fourth act of Darika's shame cycle involved a scouting part who
anticipated her being shamed and feeling shameful. In the following conversation, Darika noticed that, in addition to the gerbil who reacted to criticism and was not protecting anyone (and was therefore an exile), she had
four anxious protectors who were always on high alert. She dubbed them
her *reputation parts*. The ring leader was a monk named Lucretius.

DARIKA: Lucretius is from the Middle Ages. He has no sense of humor.
He likes keeping Yuri around because, according to him, Yuri is gay,
and men who like sex are dangerous. He says I should ignore Yuri. He
doesn't care if Yuri drinks and is an asshole because he keeps other
men away.

THERAPIST: How do you feel toward Lucretius?

DARIKA: My family is Hindu, so how weird is that? Where did he come
from? He says he wants me to be invisible.

THERAPIST: What happens when you get noticed?

[*Darika hesitates and looks at me, a European American woman, for a
few moments before answering.*]

DARIKA: I don't want to hurt your feelings, but White people can be mean.

THERAPIST: You have a part who worries about saying that to me.

DARIKA: Well, I don't like to generalize.

THERAPIST: Have you had experiences with mean White people?

DARIKA: Yeah.

THERAPIST: I'm not offended. If your parts ever feel I'm being racist or
offensive in some way, I hope they'll speak up. Will they? (*Darika
nods.*) Sounds like Lucretius anticipates trouble from men and White
people.

DARIKA: Yes.

THERAPIST: How does he protect you?

DARIKA: He keeps the sexy teenager in check. He hates teenage boys, especially White ones. He lectures me all the time about not disappointing
my parents. He warns me about everything from the risks of not smil-
ing when I'm talking to White people to crossing the road because cars
are dangerous.

THERAPIST: He tries to keep you out of trouble.

DARIKA: (*Laughs.*) And he's got these two nuns working for him. The three of them worry about everything! I think they'd like to lock me in a nunnery. . . . They're nodding.

Lucretius and the nuns had the job of anticipating trouble and getting Darika's sexy teenage part to behave. They tried to scare her and undermine her confidence. They also tried and failed to control other people, especially, at this point in her life, Yuri. As the next vignette illustrates, sooner or later rebellious parts will escalate and doom the inhibition project.

● An Example of Act 5: Shaming Others

Darika's warrior part relished being cruel and liked blaming someone else. Note that its complaints had validity. Although warrior parts don't need valid complaints, they often build on a demonstrable case, and Yuri was giving the warrior a lot of ammunition. He had refused to try couple therapy or therapy on his own; he was depressed and drinking; he seemed pleased when her young exile, who feared being alone, clung to him; he accepted her financial support; and he called her an ogre when she got angry.

DARIKA: I have this big seesaw thing with Yuri. When I come home from work and see him lying on the couch, I flip out. Then he storms around saying he'd rather be homeless than live with me—and I grovel. On Friday I begged him to stay. I literally said *I can't live without you*, which we both know is absurd.

THERAPIST: And what do you say or do before that, when you flip out?

DARIKA: Oh, anything to humiliate him. *What a loser! You're not a real man*, stuff like that. I threw my jacket at him recently. I like to see him cringe.

THERAPIST: How do you feel toward the angry part, Darika?

DARIKA: I like it.

THERAPIST: Can I talk to it directly? (*Darika nods.*) You can listen. So, I'll talk to the angry part. What do you like most about being angry?

DARIKA'S ANGRY PART: I've given him second and third chances, and he drinks all day! I'm like, wow, this is overdue! He deserves this.

THERAPIST: Do you know the Darika-who's-not-a-part?

DARIKA'S ANGRY PART: No.

THERAPIST: Okay. I'm going to talk to her again and you can listen. So, Darika, did you hear the angry part? It doesn't know who you are yet. How do you feel toward it now?

DARIKA: I guess I appreciate it. And I'm embarrassed that you should know about it.

THERAPIST: Oh, I like angry parts. I've met lots of them. What would we do without them? But they take on so much responsibility. Would everyone inside be willing to let you help your angry part? (*Darika nods.*) Would it like to meet you?

DARIKA: It's not interested in me.

THERAPIST: Okay.

DARIKA: But it would like me to listen.

THERAPIST: Is everyone else willing to let you hear from it? (*Darika nods.*) What does it want you to know?

DARIKA: If I insist on being a doormat, somebody's got to do something.

THERAPIST: So, it counters a passive part?

DARIKA: I guess. A desperate part. I think it's the gerbil. This part believes the gerbil is me (*a pause*). But wait. The gerbil protects a little girl.

THERAPIST: What if you could help her?

DARIKA: The angry one isn't going to go away.

THERAPIST: I wouldn't want it to go away. But if you were to help the gerbil and the little girl, would the angry one need to be so fierce?

DARIKA: Maybe not.

In this encounter, we see that Darika's warrior part couldn't control a needy exile and its timid protector, the gerbil. These parts were willing to let Yuri exploit her, so the angry part attacked Yuri. As the power struggle between her warrior part and Yuri's own angry protector escalated, so, too, did the risk of serious violence. If either of them had been able to garner some mental space and enough physiological regulation to pay attention internally and take care of their own vulnerability, they could have stepped out of this dangerous dynamic. But she and Yuri were not equipped to help themselves at this point—Darika could barely convince her parts to unblend a little bit in therapy sessions. At the same time, she and Yuri weren't willing to part company.

● An Example of Act 6: The Feel-Better Rescue Team

Darika's sixth act involved a reactive protector bingeing on sweets, which motivated another part to manage the risk of weight gain by restricting her food intake.

DARIKA: I'm terrified of being fat and getting diabetes like my grandmother, but I can't seem to stop eating sweets. I wake up thinking about what hour I can having something sweet. I don't eat anything except black coffee before noon. I have to do that because I'd start the day off with kheer if I let myself. My grandmother made the best kheer. This milk pudding I could eat all day long.

THERAPIST: You have parts who get comfort from kheer?

DARIKA: Some days I don't eat a meal at all, I just gobble sweet things, like kheer and dates and raisins and chocolate. I have a part who says all that is natural so it's good for me. But really, it's sugar, isn't it? It makes me feel tired.

THERAPIST: So, some parts get comfort from eating sweets, but the body feels tired and other parts worry. What would you feel if you didn't eat sweets?

DARIKA: I don't know.

THERAPIST: Is it okay to imagine not eating a sweet and see what happens?

DARIKA: Hmm. Okay (*long pause*). Anxiety builds.

THERAPIST: And then what?

DARIKA: I want to stop it.

THERAPIST: What if you could help the anxious part? (*Darika nods.*) Would it like to have help? (*Darika nods.*) Ask if it protects anyone else.

DARIKA: Yes. An anxious part.

THERAPIST: So, you have an anxious part who protects an anxious part. Is this the gerbil and the little girl? (*Darika nods.*) Who needs help first?

DARIKA: The little girl.

THERAPIST: Where do you find her?

DARIKA: She's turning away so I won't look at her. She's about 4.

THERAPIST: Is she aware of you?

DARIKA: Yes.

THERAPIST: Does she know who you are?

DARIKA: No.

THERAPIST: Would she like to meet you?

DARIKA: Yes. But she doesn't want me to come any closer.

THERAPIST: She's the boss.

DARIKA: She likes that.

THERAPIST: How do you feel toward her?

DARIKA: I'd like to know more about her.

As we discovered over time, Darika's anxious 4-year-old was an exile, a part who longed for more time with her parents, who got great comfort from her grandmother but was acutely aware of her grandmother's lack of power and confidence in the foreign world of the United States. Unlike her cheerful older brother, who seemed to gobble life up, this little girl felt needy, burdensome, and afraid.

● Acts 1 + 2: So That's What Happened!

Clients come to therapy with present-day concerns, yet we end up going into the past because something happened back then that burdened them with the beliefs and feelings that drive their current shame management strategies—those present-day concerns. But because the shaming thing that happened is emotional plutonium, we often get to it last. Darika's exile turned out to be a multi-age child. She showed Darika how lonely she had felt at home, how she had clung to her grandmother, how she had been bullied at her private school by a female White European American gym teacher whose contemptuous remarks were explicitly racist. And, finally, Darika reconnected with the tough teenage part who had turned away from her grandmother. She reminded Darika that she had been assaulted by a White European American boy after a football game at her high school when she was 14 years old. He was older, had been drinking, and was making racist and misogynist jokes during the game. She told him to shut up and later, as everyone was leaving, he punched her in the face. His friends dragged him away, and she lied to the school about her black eye because she feared the response from adults would call more attention to her in school.

THERAPIST: With all this, what did she come to believe about herself?

DARIKA: She was a throwaway.

THERAPIST: How does she feel now?

DARIKA: Well, she can feel me here.

THERAPIST: How is that?

DARIKA: Good.

THERAPIST: When she's ready, no rush, but when she's ready you can help her let go of that belief.

Witnessing can be a quick process, or it can roll out over more than one session. Its defining feature is ease. With protector resistance down and the exile's needs being met in a strong connection with the Self, what it shows or tells is often deeply personal and moving to witness. If any protectors get nervous along the way, our job is to help them proactively so the exile can continue telling its story and directing the show. We may also want to remind the exile, as I do in the preceding case, that its burdens can be released whenever it's ready.

The Shame Cycle in Brief

- *Historical shame:* A bad thing happened to me.
  - Someone shamed me.
  - Or, I felt that I didn't belong and, in an effort to help me belong, an internal critic began to shame me.
- *Agreement:* I am bad.
  - I felt shameful.
- *Instrumental (inner) shaming:* You are bad.
  - My protectors shame my exiles and my firefighters.
  - My exiles are primed to accept that judgment—they feel ashamed.
  - My firefighters work harder to distract from feeling shameful or silence critics and soothe distressed parts.
  - My protectors shame other people.
- *Recovery:* A bad thing happened to me.
  - I am compassionate, I feel loved, I reject the message of shaming.

Injured, Not Broken

Coming full circle, when a client says, "I have a problem with shame," their problem isn't only the experience of feeling shameful, it's the cycle we've just reviewed. As I mentioned, the prompting event, that initial shaming experience that came first chronologically, is likely to be revealed late in therapy. This event (or the time period covering many such events) is what protectors have been trying to undo, deny, hide, outface, and so on. In service of this goal, they have tried to conceal the evidence—the injured part who they believe caused the problem and who would surely divulge its story given the chance. We step into this delicate predicament with a bold assertion (that part is wounded, not broken, and it can heal) and with some surprising proposals about how healing happens (if you relax, someone will show up inside to facilitate). It should not surprise us if protectors need time to digest this offer.

EXERCISE

Journal

Consider these questions and write your thoughts down.

1. When bad things happen, how do you treat yourself?
   Are you kind to yourself?
   Are you critical of yourself?

Do you look for someone else to blame?

Do you plot revenge?

Do your self-critical and self-protective parts get into conflict?

2. How do you want to treat yourself?

Think of a situation in which you act like someone who loves you and imagine that playing out.

3. How do you treat other people?

Think of a situation in which you have been unkind to someone else and imagine making a repair. How does that feel?

Think of a situation in which you've been kind to someone else and imagine doing that for yourself. How does that feel?

Conclusion

What we normally call shame, as I see it, is a multi-act cycle that occurs within (and because of) the plural mind. Internal or external shamers may have good intent, but as good intent can lead to bad outcomes, intent is no way to measure the usefulness of shaming. When we shame each other, whether for the sake of improvement or to exert power, we initiate the cycle described here, with one part shaming another part and reinforcing the sense of shamefulness, which, ultimately, motivates reactive protectors to become shamelessly antisocial. We cannot shame ourselves or each other into a higher state of being.

So, let's go back where we started. Bad things happen. Children who take them to heart and believe *I am* . . . (too much, too little, defective, unfit, unworthy, wrong, and the like) get burdened with a dangerous identity. Their Self would know that the original insult was a motivated fiction, but they have no access to their Self, so the insult becomes a source of personal suffering and interpersonal conflict. Although many cultures, religions, and governing institutions are attached to the idea that shaming is a necessary tool of education and social control—that shamefulness is essential to self-inhibition—the sense of worthlessness does not produce our better nature (compassion does that), repair relationships (guilt does that), or lead us to forgive each other (kindness and mercy do that).

In therapy, we don't treat the bad thing, which is history; we reveal its underlying fiction and explore whether self-generated negative sequelae have been effective at preventing more injury. Because the protectors who create the negative sequelae have positive intentions (for us if not for others), we befriend and praise them. When they feel validated and safer, they let exiled parts tell their stories. Feeling heard and loved, exiles discard shaming beliefs about their value—at which point *I am* reverts to *it happened*.

CHAPTER 5

Empathy

So far I've offered a number of examples of how the plural model of mind can influence our view of the self-conscious emotions, shame and guilt, and how it might affect our thinking on some large recurring themes in psychotherapy: identity, change, acceptance, and psychic defiance of external pressures. The next two chapters ask how shame and guilt are relevant to ruinous but durable relational attachments. I set the table for that inquiry in this chapter by looking at how empathy and compassion function in the plural mind.

Empathy and Compassion

To feel compassion is to feel *for* others, to be concerned and willing to act on their behalf. To empathize is to feel *with* others and, when the brain is mature enough, to try to understand them in this way as well. Empathy has two stages, emotional and cognitive. Emotional empathy, the first stage, shows up in preverbal babies when one cries and other babies within earshot cry as well. That is, feelings are contagious for babies (Singer & Klimecki, 2014). By toddlerhood, as children develop a sense of *me* and *you*, they begin to have cognitive empathy in addition to emotional empathy. They engage in *perspective taking* because they are beginning to have, as researchers say, a *theory of mind* (Zahn-Waxler, Radke-Yarrow, Wagner, & Chapman, 1992). In plainer language, a toddler can feel with another person but also think about them as someone separate.

As full self-consciousness (*I'm separate and others see me*) dawns between the ages of 4 and 5 (Rochat, 2003), the child is theoretically on the way to mature empathy: *I feel with you but I'm not you.* Mature empathy promotes curiosity and forges connections, and adults who respect acts of differentiation help children develop a good measure of mature empathy and clarity about who's who in relationships. But what of children who aren't validated, don't feel seen, or get punished for being different from their caretakers? A confident, differentiated sense of self is a developmental achievement that requires a long, clear runway. Forbidding or frightening interpersonal interactions are obstacles on that runway. When an adult intrudes on a child's sense of legitimacy, the child's protectors respond by hiding vulnerable parts and concealing personal needs. How does empathy operate in a system like that?

To answer that question, let's think about the goals of the parts in different roles. In general, protectors empathize when it serves their agenda. If a manager part, for example, wanted to ensure their person's social inclusion, it would promote empathic identification with the group it deemed most desirable. If a child's manager part was handling a dangerous adult, it might want the child to empathize with that adult rather than getting angry. And the same would be true later on in life with a dangerous partner or a temperamental boss. Or, if a manager part was concerned about the self-esteem of siblings, it might use empathy to inhibit the child's competitive parts. We could spin an endless variety of valid scenarios that would involve empathy, inhibition, fear of anger, and relational loyalty.

In contrast to managers, reactive firefighter parts, who want relief now and don't care how their behavior affects other people or even their own person down the road, are generally viewed as not having interpersonal empathy. Yet in one important way they are empathic. They're exquisitely attuned to the pain of exiled parts and switch on instantly to soothe, distract, or suppress those feelings when they break into consciousness. Like soldiers who tolerate killing out of loyalty to the person standing next to them, their scope of empathy is extremely narrow, and their methods can be very costly.

If the empathy of protectors is driven by parsimonious agendas, how about the empathy of exiles? These parts live in compulsory isolation, feeling excluded and longing for rescue, so they're primed to *feel* and *identify* with vulnerability, shamefulness, and fear. For them, empathizing is a proxy route to conscious awareness and attention. But protectors are just as allergic to proxy shamefulness as they are to the homegrown variety. A protector might, for example, distract from the exile's empathy by falsely reassuring the person who feels hurt (*You're fine*), by outright denying their feelings (*You don't feel that way*), or by insisting on feeling guilty about them (*I caused you to feel bad*). Alternately, it might reject the person with whom the exile is empathizing (*I'm not like you*) or project onto them (*You be me instead of me*).

And this is just what might be occurring inside the person whose exiles are doing the empathizing. The person toward whom that empathy is directed also has parts. Their exiles also feel helpless and shameful, and their protectors are also vigilant. An observer's empathy might seem to them like a dangerous intrusion into purposely hidden feelings. In this case, they will not be happy recipients of empathy. Although protectors feel threatened by exile-to-exile empathy in some circumstances, in settings in which group cohesion is a matter of safety and survival, they may sponsor an empathic ingroup connection despite being decidedly unempathic toward the people who are affected by the group's behavior. The coup attempt in Washington, D.C., on January 6, 2021, was an interesting illustration of this phenomenon. In videos of the event, insurrectionists can be seen comforting each other and expressing concern even as they assaulted the Capitol police and threatened to kill various politicians.

A Child's Empathy

Who is responsible for whom? In the normal developmental progression, parents are responsible for their children, and then adult children gradually become responsible for their aging parents. Of necessity, the children of dysfunctional adults reverse this formula and do their best to parent their nominal caretakers. The next two chapters explore this phenomenon in depth. But parent–child relationships are relevant to the topic of empathy, so we'll broach it first with this example.

● Shira's Empathy

When we began working together, Shira was a 20-year-old, cisgender, heterosexual, Lithuanian Jewish American college student who came to therapy after a long history of anxiety, having participated in a variety of therapies. Her father had been, at times, highly critical and explosive with her since she was a toddler. She had spent years addressing this in various kinds of therapy, most recently in IFS.

Several years later, having established her independent life firmly, she reported the following interaction with her father after a visit home.

SHIRA: I was there to see an old friend and say hi to my parents. We've all gotten along very well since I got married. But out of the blue this time he came into my old bedroom where I was staying and started yelling at me. He said awful things. He blocked the doorway. He told my mother to butt out. Boy, did I feel trapped! (*Tearfully.*) It was horrible.

THERAPIST: Has he ever been violent?

SHIRA: No. This is what he does. He did it when I was little. I don't know what to do.

THERAPIST: What do you hear inside?

SHIRA: I have a part that worries about cutting off from my parents.

THERAPIST: So, there's a part who would like to cut off?

SHIRA: Yes.

THERAPIST: And a part who doesn't want to do that?

SHIRA: I'm so worried about him.

THERAPIST: Another part is worried about him?

SHIRA: Yes.

THERAPIST: Why?

SHIRA: Well, now he feels guilty. He's been apologizing. But I wonder if something is wrong with him.

THERAPIST: What about you?

SHIRA: Right.

THERAPIST: Let's help your scared, hurt part first and then we'll talk about what you might want to do.

In this segment of a session, we heard from a blended part who empathized with her father, worried about him, and wanted to protect him from feeling guilty. That is, this part wanted to protect her father from the consequences of his behavior. In the long run, the impulse to protect someone else from consequences is sure to backfire because there are consequences. When a transgressor is protected, the consequences accrue to the recipient, and eventually an angry part of the recipient takes action. If she were to set limits firmly but kindly now, her angry part probably wouldn't need to assert an extreme solution later on. Her young part's empathy was interfering with her ability to take care of her own injury, protect herself, and maintain an important relationship.

Empathy and Polarized Systems

Empathy between exiles also exacerbates protector polarizations. The #MeToo revelations of 2017 in the United States, which involved a flood of disclosures about violent misogyny on the part of powerful men, illustrate this effect at the national level. A number of high-profile male media figures responded to #MeToo by announcing that they could relate because they had wives and daughters, revealing a concern that was contingent on their ability to imagine being personally affected. They were roundly criticized for being unwilling to extend themselves toward women categorically, but I use them as an example because I don't view them as unique or particularly culpable. On the contrary, I think their behavior illustrates the universal, daily challenge empathy poses for us all.

Every day, we have to choose what we're willing to read, look at, and know about the suffering of others, human and nonhuman. Those of us

who live in cities and towns must decide how to respond to street dwellers
when we do errands. Every day all of us must choose what we'll grapple
with about the suffering of future generations and, indeed, all life on the
planet, with the catastrophe of climate change. To feel another's pain now
or imagine it in the future is to expend precious energy. Why would I volunteer to feel your pain, and why would you volunteer to feel mine?

But the fact is, we do it a lot. From what I've observed, exiled young
parts are particularly promiscuous empathizers, and protectors see the
specter of emotional overwhelm in all that vicarious pain. In the field of
mental health, we call it burnout. Clients call it a crisis. Whatever we call
it, protective parts fear, above all, being flooded with negative feelings. As
a result, they often determine eligibility for empathy according to similarity. They let us extend psychic space, understanding, and the benefit of the
doubt to people who are like us.

Sometimes this works well. There's nothing inherently wrong with
homogeneous groups. Teachers, trainers, and camp directors all do group-
forming exercises to highlight similarities and foster rapport. Identification pitches a tent for the group—by design, a small tent. And sometimes
a small tent is just right. Baseball fans choose teams and happily cheer
together. The mutual identification and exclusivity of monogamous partners is a benefit to those who choose it.

But when systems polarize around threatening issues that relate to
fairness and access to resources, a small tent can produce indifference and
cruelty toward everyone outside the tent. Groups that feel shamed are particularly at risk of protective parts taking action to disown and project
their sense of shamefulness by calling others inferior, lacking, and so on.
Even so, if external challenges were to disappear, within-group heterogene-
ity would soon emerge, with new alliances forming and new polarizations
developing.

Let's say, for example, that two very different religious communities
come into close proximity. As the communities stand in contrast, each will
be more acutely aware of what they share internally. But take the two religions out of proximity, removing that within-group pressure to conform
and cohere, and everything inside the communities will shift. Alliances will
form over similarities (*you and I were born in Ohio*), and polarities will
grow due to differences (*we like the room to be hot, you like it cold*).*
Groupings are thus forever forming and fracturing across multiple system
levels under the influence of protective parts who connect first and foremost
by identifying, which makes them parsimonious with empathy where difference is involved. If we believe the formula that former President Barack
Obama and Pope Francis endorse—*empathize and then you will identify
(and behave well)*—we miss the formula that our protective parts seem to
prefer, which is *identify and then empathize.*

---

* See, for example, Roubein and Shammas (2022).

Intervene in Internal Battles

Have a journal handy to take notes. Think of someone you really dislike. Be honest, you're not going to tell anyone else. It can be someone you know well or not.

Step One

- Notice your body:
  - Disgust?
  - Shrinking?
  - Physical discomfort?
  - An urge to think about something else?
- Now think of something you dislike about yourself.
  - Note that this means one of your parts (or a group of parts) is judging another one of your parts.
- Ask the judging part (or parts) if they would relax back and let you extend some curiosity to the part they dislike.
- If so, continue to Step Two.
- If not, don't argue, but do ask why and write down what you hear in a journal.

Step Two

- How do you feel toward this disliked part?
  - If you notice the negative feelings of other parts, ask them to relax so you can hear from the target part.
    - If they refuse, don't argue, but do ask why and write down what you hear in a journal.
  - If they agree, notice how you feel toward the target part (the disliked part) now.
- When it's okay to be curious, ask the target part to notice you. Then ask it these questions and write down the answers:
  - Do you protect anyone?
    - If not, this part is an exile. Put it in a safe place and set the intention to return when you have checked for permission from protective parts at a later time.
    - If so, proceed. Ask: *What would happen if you stopped doing what you do?* and write down what you hear.
      - If it names another protector (*I would watch too much TV*), ask if it's okay to talk with that part, too, and invite it to join you.
      - Then ask the other protector the same question: *What would happen if you stopped doing what you do?*
      - Once you've heard from both parts, ask this question: *If I could help the part (or parts) you protect, would you need to be this extreme?*
    - Write down what you hear and thank them.

Now you know two protectors who are in conflict because they have different views on how to protect an exile (or two different exiles), who will be able
to stand down when you help the exile(s). Use this information as a road map for
further inquiry and get permission to help the exile(s).

The Role of Compassion

My point about empathy is that we blind ourselves to its risks if we expect
only benefits. Which brings us to the Self. Well-differentiated, non-self-
interested empathy is, in my view, a sign that we have access to our Self—
not because the Self is empathic but because when the Self is available, parts
don't have to navigate the potential pitfalls of empathy alone. Several years
ago, Matthieu Ricard, a monk who is an expert meditator, participated in a
brain-imaging empathy study led by empathy researcher Tania Singer. After
watching a video on the intensely traumatic lives of children in a Roma-
nian orphanage, Ricard empathized with the children for 2 hours while his
brain was scanned. Singer then offered to take a break before scanning him
during a compassion meditation. He declined to take a break because he
was finding the suffering unbearable and wanted to switch to compassion
immediately to "soak" that suffering in loving-kindness (Mindful Living
Community, 2021).

Illustrating that empathy and compassion are not on a functional continuum, and that so-called compassion fatigue would be more accurately
called empathy fatigue, the imaging from this study showed neural pain
pathways lighting up in Ricard's brain when he empathized and pleasure
pathways lighting up when he practiced loving-kindness compassion. While
the research world has absorbed and disseminated this news (Klimecki,
Leiberg, Lamm, & Singer, 2013; Klimecki, Leiberg, Ricard, & Singer,
2014; Klimecki, Ricard, & Singer, 2013; Klimecki & Singer, 2012; Singer
& Klimecki, 2014), it has not yet been fully digested by mental health pro-
viders nor has it percolated far into popular thinking. Regardless, Singer's
finding is highly relevant for our purposes.

From the IFS perspective, compassion and love are the purest expression of what we call Self-energy. They are mutually exclusive with shaming,
and they heal the aftereffects of attachment disruption and trauma. When
prosecutorial critics hand vulnerable parts a life sentence, the Self com-
mutes it and pardons the critics; when firefighter parts engage in destructive extremes, it forgives them and takes responsibility for their behavior;
when exiled parts believe they are unlovable, it begs to differ. The Self
says, "I see you, I want to know you, I'm concerned, and I will act on your
behalf." Nowhere does it say, "I have to be you in order to care about you."

Identification is a potent but narrow formula for maintaining relationships. In truth, we don't have to be the same to care for each other,

and, ironically, identification can be a major challenge for two people who exile similar parts. Protective parts are too close to exiles, too much in agreement with their devastating beliefs to help them. In contrast, the Self doesn't identify with the exile and doesn't share its fear or its feeling of being shameful. Because the Self is not a part, it's not caught up in the affective web that parts weave by feeling with each other. Instead, the Self has compassion and feels *for* parts, and Singer's study shows how this looks in the brain.

Whether in individual, couple, or family therapy, IFS aims to give emotionally interwoven parts permission to differentiate and be themselves. The motto is *All parts are welcome!* Just as a comfortably differentiated couple is better at navigating the challenges of intimacy, parts are better at handling their empathic emotional involvement with one another when they don't have to agree, when they don't have to do anything to or for each other in order to be accepted and loved. Anxiety about who will be acknowledged, seen, and have legitimacy subsides when no one is banished. The Self's inclusive welcome gives each part permission to be. In the words of one of my clients, "If my parts can feel me, they don't need to jump on me. If I am able to feel them, they don't need to fight over who gets felt."

Can We Be Different and Safe with Each Other?

To feel differentiated, accepted, and included is an ideal. Clients don't start at that ideal, of course, but therapists have (in theory at least) given themselves a head start and can function as a guide. If someone who is different from me chooses me for therapy, it is my job to be their guide. I'm a cisgender, heterosexual, English Scottish American female who speaks just one language. Let's say a male, transgender, first-generation Mexican American client who speaks both English and Spanish comes to me for therapy. To serve him well enough, I need to know and use the preferred vocabulary of the transgender community, I need to be educated about the physical and social challenges he may have faced or be facing, I need to listen and learn about his experience, I need to be curious about his culture of origin, and I need to have compassion for him—feel for him, care about him, understand and validate his feelings, and be willing to act on his behalf should the need arise. Singer's research tells us that compassion and empathy are distinct phenomena in the brain. In theory, I can do all that for him without feeling his pain or identifying with him.

Of course, in practice I will feel his pain. I have parts, and parts are prolific empathizers. We can't (and shouldn't in my view) try to keep parts from having empathy for each other or for the parts of other people. But part-to-part empathy comes with risks. Good enough access to the Self can mitigate but not eliminate the risks we face when parts take over. If a client's pain activates pain in my brain and my parts respond by making assumptions based on my experience, I'll miss what matters to my client. But if my empathizing parts separate so that my Self is available, their empathy will become background to the foreground of my curiosity and concern. My job is not to ask *How are you similar to me?* but *What happened to you?*

Practice Compassion

In general, you can help your parts unblend by noticing them and getting curious. To practice compassion, notice the shoes they're in and feel *for* them. Take notes.

1. Find a part with important feelings. This is your target part.

2. Ask the target part to separate from you and explain its mission (if it has one) and its needs. As the target part communicates, notice if you feel *for* it (compassion) or *with* it (empathy).

3. If you are empathizing (feeling with the target part), ask your empathizing part(s) to separate. If they are willing to dial down the level at which they share their feelings with you, they can go on empathizing without interfering.

4. Return to the target part and notice how you feel toward it now. If, for some reason, compassion is beyond reach, ask inside if it's okay for you to start by being curious about the target part.

5. When you have permission, listen to the target part.

6. Ask the target part to explain who, if anyone, it protects. If it's not a protector, it is an exile. Feel *for* the part (have compassion) as it answers. Invite the part to notice that you are different. You are not a part, which is why you can help.

7. Take time to extend compassion and loving-kindness to the target part.

8. What happens in you when you feel compassion?

9. What happens in your relationship with the part (or person) for whom you feel compassion?

Conclusion

Physical and emotional pain form a necessary proactive alarm system. We're at great risk if we never feel pain. For example, people with leprosy are inexorably nibbled away by contact with their environment because their nerve endings are numb. The same is true for people who dissociate a great deal. When all is well, we feel pain, and it tells us what to avoid, what to take care of, and so on—and it turns off. When it doesn't turn off, we get a cascade of the kinds of protective strategies and negative consequences I've been describing in this book, which should give us caution about oversimplifying or generalizing the beneficial role of empathy in human systems. When an internal system is dominated by the likes of wall parts (who show up as literal walls and block access to exiles or information about the past), dissociative parts, compliant parts, angry parts, narcissistic parts, intransigent nonverbal parts, and so on, it pays to remember that they take on these roles in order to banish emotional pain that doesn't turn off, and they can't be expected to welcome more pain. Yet to empathize with pain is to feel pain.

Empathy thus poses a Goldilocks dilemma for mental health treatment. We can have too much or too little empathy for our clients, our clients can have too much or too little empathy for the people in their lives, and a client's parts can have too much or too little empathy for each other. Too much empathy motivates protectors to suppress feelings, whereas too little signals that protectors have already shut feelings down. But empathy itself is neither a culprit nor a cure-all. We don't need our parts to have less empathy, and we couldn't make that happen anyway. What we do need is for our parts to separate and welcome the Self. To give our parts internal stability, we need, as Singer's research tells us, a good blueprint for accessing compassion.

When exiled parts feel legitimatized by the Self's embrace, they can let their fears and shamefulness go and stop overloading the internal system with personal and vicarious pain. In turn, protectors can stop fusing with suffering caretakers or projecting feared emotions onto others. All our parts can feel welcome and be free. But as we aim for this outcome, we must remember that parts don't liberate each other. Even when protectors are mortally divided among themselves over how to be safe, they can agree that vulnerable parts who get hurt are shameful and need to be exiled. When it is alone, functioning without leadership from the Self, the system of parts lacks a necessary counterbalance. The unity of opposites between parts and the Self creates balance. With this in mind, I'll repeat the simple, user-friendly formula I've developed in my therapy practice. Parts feel pain. Sometimes it's their pain, and sometimes the pain originated with someone else. Either way, when they feel pain, they need help. The Self, which is fully aware of their pain and feels compassion, is there to help. Our ticket to freedom isn't empathy between parts, it's the Self's love and compassion for all parts.

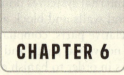

CHAPTER 6

Shame-Based Trauma Bonding
The Child Who Shares Shamefulness

Clients will often explain their devotion to a harming caretaker by citing wishes and worries, such as a need for love, a longing for connection, and the fear of being abandoned and alone. Such wishes speak of dependency and are typical of the exiled parts we find in adult clients. On the other hand, clients also cite feelings and worries that are more typical of protectors, such as pity or the desire to avoid future guilt, illustrating that a client's self-sacrifice can be animated by either exiles or protectors. When children are loyal and self-sacrificing with adults who neglect or harm them, I call it *trauma bonding*. In this chapter, I cite examples of some convoluted relational scenarios involving loyalty, self-sacrifice, and projection that illustrate trauma bonding and the importance of tracking the client's experience without judgment, which is to say with curiosity. Although trauma bonding isn't a sticking point for all clients, it's something to consider when a client isn't getting traction or relief in therapy.

The first example illustrates a grown son and his father sorting out the origin and disparate meanings of a shared water phobia. The second is the inquiry of a rape survivor into her feelings, loyalties, and desire for vindication. The third is an adult in group therapy realizing that her internal system has formed a unilateral bond with another group member that features a mix of identification and revulsion. All three examples illustrate a strategy IFS calls the *U-turn*. By guiding the client to turn their attention inside, the U-turn aims to bring the client's attention to protective parts who are trying to undo what's been done, project qualities they dislike, and so on. The U-turn is an invaluable tool for helping protective parts to unblend.

Examples of Sharing Shamefulness

● Ben + Lucas: *I'll Be You with You*

Lucas came to therapy to explore his water phobia and then invited his father, Ben, who was also afraid of water, to come for a joint session. In the chronology of this therapy, I met first with the son, Lucas. As the following vignette reveals, Lucas felt an adult need to get over a water phobia, but his young protectors were attached to the phobia out of loyalty to his father.

LUCAS: My fiancée loves to swim, so I thought I should try to get over this water thing.

THERAPIST: Is anyone else in your family afraid of water?

LUCAS: My father.

THERAPIST: Do you know why?

LUCAS: (*Shrugs.*) Some childhood thing. We always went to the desert for vacations. No problem for me. I love the desert!

[*His lack of curiosity suggests awareness of his father's emotional fragility on this subject.*]

THERAPIST: How do you feel toward the part of you who fears water?

LUCAS: I guess I just picked it up.

[*He doesn't answer my question.*]

THERAPIST: Would there be a problem with you not fearing water?

[*I try a different tack.*]

LUCAS: I don't know how to swim.

[*Again, he doesn't answer my question.*]

THERAPIST: If you could swim and be safe in water, would any part of you object to swimming?

[*I jump over his practical objection with a hypothetical question.*]

LUCAS: I hear, *Yes.* But why?

THERAPIST: Would that part be willing to say why?

LUCAS: I hear, *What about Dad?*

THERAPIST: What about Dad?

LUCAS: He'd be alone.

THERAPIST: So, you have a part who takes care of your father.

LUCAS: I guess.

THERAPIST: And what does it believe about you?

LUCAS: I'm a good person. I can't leave him alone.

After this session, Lucas became curious about the origin of his father's water phobia and invited Ben to a session. The following snippet, which begins after Ben has connected with an 8-year-old exile, is from the middle of that father–son session.

BEN: He watched his brother drown.

THERAPIST: What was that like for him?

BEN: He stood there.

[*He names an act rather than a feeling, indicating that the boy froze in that moment, which, after the fact, became central to Ben's identity.*]

THERAPIST: What was the worst thing about him freezing in that moment?

BEN: He didn't help his brother.

THERAPIST: And, so, what did he come to believe about himself?

BEN: He's bad.

The hidden personal meaning of Ben's water phobia is *I am a bad person.* In contrast, the hidden personal meaning of the water phobia for Lucas is *I am a good, loyal person.* The father views himself as a relational hazard, the son as a relational gift. One generation's excruciating pain and secret identity underpins the next generation's loyalty-based bond and positive self-esteem. The literal belief—water is dangerous—has completely different personal and relational meanings for these two.

As we see in this example, a loyalty burden does not mark who *I* am the way a personal burden does. Rather, it marks who *we* are: We are anxious, we are stifled, we are doomed, we are afraid, we are outraged, and so on. Manager parts tend to take on a caretaker's burden with a mix of concern for the caretaker (*you* needs) and fear that the child would be exiled if they were to act on *me* needs. But even when a child mimics an adult's shame-based behavior or words, their underlying sense of concern is prosocial and relational rather than rooted in self-loathing. To feel connected and safe, a child's managers will comply with a caretaker's agenda and join them to have *we* beliefs. Emotionally and energetically, trying to rescue someone you need (and maybe love) is the opposite of hiding because you believe no one could love you.

● Amarie: *I Don't Want to Be You*

Amarie, a 25-year-old cisgender, heterosexual, single, mixed-race (Latinx and Indigenous) woman, was raped by a work colleague named Gavin. She was now a witness for the prosecution at his trial. The outcome would determine whether he went to prison or got his job back. Amarie was not optimistic. She was job hunting and thinking about what she wanted in advance of whatever actually happened. At the outset of this session, she was pondering what to make of his behavior, as she often did in therapy.

AMARIE: Why me?

THERAPIST: What answer do you hear?

AMARIE: He wanted to crush me. But we barely knew each other.

THERAPIST: And what do you hear about that?

AMARIE: (*Shrugs.*) I don't know. I was like . . . the opposite of him, friendly, spontaneous, no special enemies at work.

THERAPIST: And now?

AMARIE: I'm unspontaneous and untrusting and everyone avoids me. So now I'm like him.

THERAPIST: Would the parts who are now unspontaneous and untrusting like your help?

[*Suggesting a U-turn.*]

AMARIE: It was like—to me—it was like he was possessed. And now I'm the one who's possessed.

[*She ignores my question.*]

THERAPIST: Possessed by what?

AMARIE: Anger and shame, I guess.

THERAPIST: Do your parts want to carry his anger and shame?

AMARIE: No!

THERAPIST: We could help them.

[*Suggesting a U-turn.*]

AMARIE'S ANGRY PROTECTOR: No.

THERAPIST: How come?

AMARIE'S ANGRY PROTECTOR: He should feel ashamed!

THERAPIST: You have a part who wants Gavin to feel ashamed.

AMARIE'S ANGRY PROTECTOR: Of course.

THERAPIST: When someone tosses you a hot potato like shamefulness— and you can't just give it back—what do your parts do?

[*Trying for a U-turn.*]

AMARIE'S ANGRY PROTECTOR: I want him to feel what I feel! He sits in court like a zombie.

THERAPIST: And when you see him being a zombie, how do you feel?

AMARIE'S ANGRY PROTECTOR: Weak, offended, hopeless, angry.

[*This is the U-turn.*]

THERAPIST: Who is taking care of the weak, offended part? Could Amarie do that?

[*I switch to speaking to the angry part directly and press for continuing with the U-turn.*]

AMARIE'S ANGRY PROTECTOR: (*Shakes her head no.*) He has to take it back!

THERAPIST: Take what back?

AMARIE'S ANGRY PROTECTOR: That I deserved it.

THERAPIST: Do you have parts who say you deserved it?

[*Guiding Amarie back toward the U-turn.*]

AMARIE'S ANGRY PROTECTOR: Why else would it happen?

THERAPIST: Why else would it happen?

AMARIE: Okay. I see what you mean. But that's what I believe.

THERAPIST: You have a part who believes you deserved to be raped?

AMARIE: It says I never learn. I'm naive.

THERAPIST: Do you have a naïve part?

[*If a protector accuses the client of a certain behavior, it's safe to assume they're naming another part.*]

AMARIE: (*Looks out the window.*) In high school I went to a college party, drank the roofied punch, and woke up on the floor without any pants. I never told anyone. I was lucky not to get sick or pregnant. But (*leaning forward*) did I learn? Why would I do Gavin any favors? I never liked him. When he asked me to pick up some papers for work because he had a dental appointment, I said yes, but I was in a hurry. But when he opened the door, he didn't have any papers in his hand. He asked me to come inside, and this voice in my head yelled, *No!* But I went in.

THERAPIST: If you could help the part who went in, would your other parts feel safer?

AMARIE: They hate her.

[*Amarie names an inner polarity between a compliant part and parts who fear and dislike the compliant part.*]

THERAPIST: I know they can't help her, but would they let you help her? (*Amarie leans back, thinks, and then nods.*) Are you seeing her now? (*Amarie nods.*) Would she like your help? (*Amarie nods.*) Does anyone object to you helping her now? (*Amarie shakes her head no.*) How do you feel toward her?

AMARIE: I wish she wasn't so stupid.

THERAPIST: Would all the parts who want to call her names be willing to relax and let you help her? (*Amarie nods.*) How do you feel toward her now?

AMARIE: I would like to help her.

THERAPIST: Does she want your help? (*Amarie nods.*) Does she protect anyone?

AMARIE: My mother.

THERAPIST: In what way?

AMARIE: She looks for the good in people.

THERAPIST: And how does that protect your mother?

AMARIE: That's my mother. If I don't like someone, she tells me I'm confused. This part sounds just like Mom.

THERAPIST: Is she your mom?

AMARIE: No.

THERAPIST: Would it be a problem if she were different from your mom?

AMARIE: I think so. She's showing me how Mom looked when Grandpa teased her. He lived with us. He was mad when she got born again. She laughed when he teased, but I could see it hurt.

THERAPIST: So, this part protects your mother from her father? (*Amarie nods.*) How old is she?

AMARIE: Five.

THERAPIST: I see. Is everyone still willing to let you help her? (*Amarie nods.*)

● *One Week Later*

Amarie did help the 5-year-old, and the next week she had a conversation with some inner critics who were concerned about her family's reaction to the rape trial.

AMARIE: They all think I want revenge. What I really want is exoneration.

THERAPIST: Does it feel like you're the one on trial?

AMARIE: (*Considers.*) Yes.

THERAPIST: Inside as well as out?

AMARIE: Yes.

THERAPIST: You have inner critics prosecuting you?

AMARIE: Yes. And so are the people in the courtroom. And so is my family. The trial will end, but my family won't stop.

THERAPIST: How do you know?

AMARIE: They're religious.

THERAPIST: So?

AMARIE: Women have to be responsible.

THERAPIST: They blame you for his actions?

AMARIE: No, they blame *me* for my actions.

THERAPIST: I see. Would your parts agree that your family is being unfair? (*Amarie nods.*) How do you treat yourself when others treat you badly?

[*Guiding Amarie toward the U-turn again.*]

AMARIE: Some get mad, others want me to stop being the bad girl. But this really loud part wants Gavin to feel how I feel.

THERAPIST: Which is?

AMARIE: Humiliated.

THERAPIST: Are your parts open to hearing from me about that? (*Amarie nods.*) Okay. You have no power to make Gavin admit that he's guilty or that he has a part who felt ashamed before he did this or anything else. If you stay attached to that outcome, you will stay frustrated and angry. Do your parts get what I'm saying?

[*Clarifying the need for a U-turn.*]

AMARIE: Yes. But they feel sad.

THERAPIST: Would they be willing to meet you? (*Amarie raises an eyebrow.*) You helped that naive 5-year-old who protected her mother. Did they notice? (*Amarie nods.*) Would they let you help the part who was hurt by Gavin?

[*Asking permission.*]

AMARIE: They want justice. How can I help with that?

THERAPIST: What happens to the hurt part when they focus on justice?

AMARIE: She hides.

THERAPIST: Do they see? While they seek justice, or try to change the past, or work to pacify your family she's alone. We're not asking them to help her. But you can. Will they let you?

AMARIE: Yes.

Over the course of therapy Amarie's protectors kept trying to undo reality with counterfactual fantasies. They warned her not to go into Gavin's apartment, they fantasized that he would confess his guilt in court, and one loud voice insisted that justice could only be served if he felt ashamed. Like all undoing thoughts, these thoughts were the prologue for a trip to nowhere. The part who fed her the fantasy of Gavin shaming himself into contrition (feeling guilt) illustrates a common misunderstanding about shaming. It won't be a brake on rage, because it's the gas pedal. In contrast, I was urging her to pay attention to her experience, which, admittedly, is a tough sell after rape or any assault. But it is a route to relief if parts will unblend. Although she couldn't force Gavin to feel ashamed—or, more appropriately, guilty—she could release her system from feeling responsible for his behavior and shameful as a result of it.

When a bad thing happens, we either act or we freeze. Afterward, we notice our feelings, and we start thinking. We ask and answer questions. *How could you?* and *Who are you?* are common questions. *Why me?* is extremely common. When an exile asks *Why me?* managers often answer *Because . . .* and fill in the blank with particulars that can be summed up as either *you're too much* or *you're too little*. If we have sufficient external support (or perhaps a bold temperament), we may not go in that direction. Resilient people are not mysteriously immune to fear in the face of danger or to feeling hurt if an insult lands on a vulnerable spot. They don't draw the same toxic conclusions from bad experiences. Interactions can rend an attachment, but meaning creates the burden that outlasts the experience. Exiles and the parts who protect them construct personal burdens from the raw material of shaming, whereas protectors who feel guilty inhabit other peoples' burdens like hermit crabs.

Amarie was vulnerable to this trauma because of a young part who empathized and identified with her mother and made a point of trusting without justification and against the better judgment of Amarie's other parts. But I'd be remiss if I didn't add a caveat regarding rape. Although categories of transgression have common elements, each one is unique. Women can be attacked on the street by men they don't know, in the apartments of men they barely know, or at home in intimate relationships. I'm not aiming to generalize from Amarie's experience. Rather, I have illustrated two points that are important for therapy: (1) when a child feels obliged to protect their caretaker, immature decision making accrues predictably negative results and (2) a U-turn is the best first step even when a client has been victimized and needs to strategize how to be safe in the future.

● Louisa: *You Be Me Instead of Me*

Protective parts can try to rid us of shamefulness in a group setting by denying the feeling inside and projecting it onto someone else (*You be me instead of me*). Louisa, a 44-year-old, cisgender, Slovenian American woman, was attending a support group to get help quitting a long-standing tobacco habit. The group was heterogeneous in all ways except for the common goal of quitting smoking. In group, Louisa quickly developed strong feelings about one other participant, a sad, middle-aged, low-income, European American mother like her. Louisa's exiles resonated with this woman, and in response her protectors criticized the woman for all the things they criticized in Louisa. And then they complained about her in individual therapy.

LOUISA'S CRITIC: Nobody likes this person.

THERAPIST: What do you not like about her?

LOUISA'S CRITIC: She pities herself. She wants the limelight. She's selfish and greedy.

THERAPIST: You have a part who dislikes all that in her.

LOUISA'S CRITIC: I do.

THERAPIST: How do you feel toward that part.

LOUISA'S CRITIC: I think it's right.

THERAPIST: So you're seeing this woman through the eyes of a part who dislikes her. Would that part be willing to separate and see her through your eyes?

LOUISA'S CRITIC: Who are you talking about?

THERAPIST: When I say you could see this woman through your eyes I mean you, the Louisa-who's-not-a-part.

LOUISA'S CRITIC: I don't know who that is.

THERAPIST: Okay. Are you the part who dislikes this woman in the group?

[*I switch and speak with Louisa's critic directly.*]

LOUISA'S CRITIC: Yes.

THERAPIST: Would you like to meet the Louisa-who's-not-a-part?

LOUISA'S CRITIC: No.

THERAPIST: Would you be willing to meet her?

LOUISA'S CRITIC: Yes.

THERAPIST: Okay. I'll talk to her. So, Louisa, this part is willing to meet you. Ask it to look you in the eye and let you know who it sees there. (*After a silence, Louisa nods.*) Who does it see?

[*This technique, which I call* eye contact,* *is often very handy.*]

LOUISA: It's not impressed.

THERAPIST: Who's there?

LOUISA: A mousy kid.

THERAPIST: And how does the critical part feel toward the mousy kid?

LOUISA: Pities her.

THERAPIST: Ask the mousy kid to sit next to you, and then ask the critic to look again. (*Louisa nods.*) Who does it see now?

LOUISA: A grown-up.

_____

* Mike Elkin, an IFS lead trainer, created the eye-contact technique.

THERAPIST: What kind of grown-up?

LOUISA: A smart one.

THERAPIST: That's you. Would it be willing to look at the mousy kid through your eyes? (*Louisa nods.*) Who does it see now?

LOUISA: An unhappy little kid.

THERAPIST: We'll come back to this little kid. But first, would the critic be willing to look at the woman from your Smoke Enders group through your eyes?

LOUISA: Okay. Not so happy about that. But okay.

THERAPIST: Who does it see?

LOUISA: A sad lady.

THERAPIST: What's that like for the critic?

LOUISA: It liked being critical better.

THERAPIST: How come?

LOUISA: (*Chuckles.*) It's easier.

THERAPIST: Who does the critic protect?

LOUISA: The mousy kid.

THERAPIST: Would the critic like you to help the mousy kid?

LOUISA'S CRITIC: She can't be helped.

THERAPIST: Hmm. Would you be open to a little thought experiment? (*Louisa looks skeptical.*) I'll describe it. You say *I am* . . . and then say whatever comes to mind to describe this woman in the group.

[*This is a U-turn exercise.*]

LOUISA: (*After a pause.*) You think I'm like her?

THERAPIST: I don't know, but I suspect your critic thinks so.

LOUISA: (*Shrugs.*) I'm not like her.

THERAPIST: Okay.

LOUISA'S CRITIC: (*Looks at the therapist.*) Don't judge me.

THERAPIST: Have you felt judged by me? (*Louisa shakes her head no.*) If you ever feel judged, please let me know. We'll stop right away and check it out.

LOUISA: (*slowly*) Okay. I'm selfish, greedy, needy. . . . (*Makes a face.*) I do say that to myself.

THERAPIST: Your critical part says that to you. Who is it talking about?

LOUISA: The mousy kid.

[*She lapses into silence.*]

THERAPIST: Can you see her?

LOUISA: She wants attention so bad and she's so . . . blah. Nothing special. Her older sister is prettier, her younger sister is smarter. I feel for her.

THERAPIST: What do you feel for her?

LOUISA: Sad.

THERAPIST: Pity or concern?

LOUISA: Concern.

THERAPIST: The critical part calls her selfish, greedy, needy.

LOUISA: It thinks she's like. . . . Well, it's just mean to her.

THERAPIST: What does it say?

LOUISA: She's a turd.

THERAPIST: That is mean. Would it be willing to let you help her? (*She nods.*) What does she need from you?

LOUISA: She's crying. She just wants to be included.

THERAPIST: What do you say to her?

LOUISA: If you keep wanting to be someone else, you're not gonna notice anything so great about you.

THERAPIST: Does she get that?

LOUISA: Hmmm. I think she's getting the idea. She came over for a hug.

When Louisa's sad young part empathized and identified with another woman's sad part in a therapy group, Louisa's critic put the kibosh on the connection by trashing the other woman just as it habitually trashed her sad little girl part inside. When people prescribe empathy to polarized systems, their unspoken assumption is: *You will benefit from treating each other the way you treat yourselves.* But if we scorn, dismiss, deny, ignore, smother, drug, or otherwise silence and distract from some of our parts, others won't benefit from being treated in the same way. As we see with Louisa, empathy between exiles can cause trouble. Protectors don't bring more openness, care, consideration, and kindness to other people's exiles than to their own. The more we've been hurt, the more our protectors abhor vulnerability.

EXERCISE

Do a U-Turn to Help Your Exiles

In this exercise, you will do a U-turn. Of course, a U-turn is easier to do in moments of calm than in moments of stress, which is why it's good to practice and develop a habit of viewing protector reactivity as a signal to find the exile. To notice how your parts usually react to insults, ask yourself this question: *When I feel hurt, how do I treat myself?*

- Does a part:
  - Copy the shamer and shame you?
  - Tell you how to improve?
  - Get mad at the other person and defend you?
  - Distract with substances, food, sex, TV, or some other firefighter activity?
  - Collapse into despair or depression?
  - Feel nauseous?
  - Want to run away?
  - Plot revenge?
  - Other?
- When protectors get active, what happens to the part who got hurt?
- Ask your protectors for permission to help the part who got hurt. How do they respond?
- Notice how you feel toward the part who got hurt.
- Check to be sure you have enough Self-energy and then ask the part who got hurt what it needs from you. Thank it. Take notes and return to this part.

Conclusion

We can share another person's feelings voluntarily (*I'll be you with you*), we can feel forced to feel with another person (*I have to be you with you*), and we can try to coerce another person to feel a feeling that we want to deny (*You be me instead of me*). Joining, recruiting, expelling, swapping—these are some of the strategies that protectors use to handle the pain of a shameful identity. These strategies create what I'm calling trauma bonds. There is always a cost for both of the people involved, and in therapy we treat people on each side of this equation.

In this chapter, we've seen shamed-based trauma bonds that formed in three different ways. A father shared a shame-based belief with his son (*you be me with me*), and his son's loyal willingness transformed (for the son) the emotional valence of his father's belief. A woman struggled with self-loathing after being traumatically injured and shamed (*I have to be you with you*). And a woman's exiles empathized and identified with another woman in a group (*I'll be you with you*), which, in turn, caused her protectors to judge and criticize the other woman (*you be me instead of me*). In the next chapter, I look at guilt-based bonds and the costs that accrue when a caretaker's protectors coerce a child into becoming the parent.

CHAPTER 7

Guilt-Based Trauma Bonding
The Child Who Takes Responsibility

Up to now we've seen proactive manager protectors who try to shame away the pain of feeling shameful and also reactive firefighter parts who distract the shamed mind or soothe the shamed body as it oscillates between alarm and shutdown. But parts who sacrifice a child's personal welfare for the interests of a caretaker belong in a different category. They start off aiming to do something beneficial for the internal system and hoping for a fair swap (I'll take care of you so you'll take care of me), but as the caretaker's protectors recruit them further into the job, the caretaker's interests become paramount. Family therapists call this child parentified; we'll talk about parentified parts.

The parentified part wants some real parenting for exiles inside (and also for siblings if they exist). On the job, it will treat the nominal caretaker like a child, anticipating needs, organizing, managing moods, and taking care not to compete or disappoint, as Karlen Lyons-Ruth demonstrated in her remarkable prospective study on attachment styles (Khoury et al., 2019; Lyons-Ruth & Brumariu, 2021). A parentified young part will do things like tamping down personal ambition, failing at something when necessary to avoid surpassing the caretaker, or silencing exuberant parts if the caretaker is depressed. In short, parentified parts will act against the wishes and interests of their own tribe and body because they're bonded to a dysfunctional caretaker by longing, fear, pity, genuine concern, and maladaptive guilt.

Clues to Parentification

Certain clues point toward the client having been recruited to parent their caretakers early in life, including the client's (1) describing a pattern of caretaking, self-sacrifice, and guilt in their adult relationships; (2) expressing empathy for (and possibly identification with) a dysfunctional caretaker, boss, or partner when one might reasonably expect them to feel angry instead; (3) expressing guilt about a developmental achievement or some other success; (4) expressing fear about disappointing other people; (5) revealing fears or prejudices that don't easily relate to their lived experience; and (6) discovering that some burdens stick around even after being released by the exile.

Clues to Parentification

The parentified part can be seen in a person who:

- Has a history of self-sacrifice along with a bent for (and some pointed rebellion against) caretaking.
  - For example, adult clients may speak of a living parent as if they are the child, or speak of being angry with the parent while meticulously caring for them.
- Has empathy for (and maybe identification with) a dysfunctional caretaker, boss, or partner where one might reasonably expect anger.
- Feels guilty about achieving developmental milestones (separation guilt) or being successful (survivor guilt).
- Hates to disappoint others.
- Has fears and biases that don't match their life experience.
- Has burdens that stick around even after being released by the exile.

Maggie: Clues to Her Parentification

Maggie was an 18-year-old, cisgender, heterosexual, Irish American high school student. Her one older brother, Jackson, lived a few states away, and her parents were divorced. She lived with her mother, Irene, and came to therapy after Irene had given her an ultimatum (therapy or move out) due to an argument over Irene's boyfriend, Craig, whom Maggie disliked intensely. Irene, in turn, disliked Maggie's friends. Maggie had considered moving out rather than going to therapy, but her parentified part would not allow it. You see, Maggie took care of Irene, cleaning the house and using money she earned on weekends to buy food, put gas in the car, and take her mother's cat to the vet. While she scoffed at Irene's disciplinary efforts and got enraged when Irene tried to exert control over her, her caretaking part never flagged. I break this example down into segments and index each segment to one of the clues mentioned above that reveal parentified parts.

● *Maggie's Parentified Part Scorns Irene*

In this monologue, Maggie's parentified part, who was blended, disparaged Irene's boyfriend and spoke of Irene as if she were the child and Maggie the parent.

MAGGIE: This asshole freakin' empties our refrigerator and watches TV all day in our house. You know what? She won't admit it but that's his pay for sticking around. She's pitiful. As soon as I finish school, I'm outta here. I'm done cleaning up after her. She better not come to me for money, either. I won't support her.

● *Maggie Has Polarized Protectors*

In this interchange, Maggie described being angry with Irene and taking care of her, revealing a polarity between a rebellious part and the parentified part.

MAGGIE: I came home from basketball practice and they were dead drunk on the floor. The kitchen was a mess, the cat was starved, the windows were wide open, and it was pouring rain. I almost took her car and drove to Colorado to live with Jackson.

THERAPIST: What did you do?

MAGGIE: (*Sighs.*) Whaddya think? I closed the windows, mopped the floor, fed the cat, did the dishes, and turned off the TV. But I didn't cover them with blankets. Fuck them.

● *Maggie's Legacy Burden of Bias*

In this exchange, Maggie spoke disparagingly about a transgender boy in her class, revealing that her parts had signed on to Irene's open bias about transgender people.

MAGGIE: He gives me the creeps. I mean your sex is your sex, right? You're born one way or the other, you don't get to choose.

THERAPIST: That's how transgender people feel.

MAGGIE: But they are choosing!

THERAPIST: Have you ever talked with someone who's transgender?

MAGGIE: I only know this one kid. She—he—used to try to be friends with me. But I just couldn't. It was too weird.

THERAPIST: A part told you that he was weird or the situation was weird?

MAGGIE: All of it. I guess that's a part.

THERAPIST: What was it concerned would happen if it didn't tell you that this boy was weird?

MAGGIE: (*After a pause, in a more subdued tone.*) I might be friends with him.

THERAPIST: And then what?

MAGGIE: Irene already thinks my friends are freaks.

THERAPIST: What does Irene say about transgender people?

MAGGIE: (*Hesitates.*) She says they're disgusting.

THERAPIST: So, if you had a transgender friend . . .

MAGGIE: (*Looks down.*) I'd never tell her. I'd never let that person anywhere near our house. I'd never be seen in public with that person in case she found out.

THERAPIST: Who would you be protecting?

MAGGIE: Irene isn't a bad person, you know. She can be mean, but that's just how she grew up.

THERAPIST: A part protects Irene? (*Maggie nods reluctantly.*) Is it afraid of Irene? (*Maggie nods.*) Does that make sense to you, Maggie?

MAGGIE: (*Sadly.*) Yes.

THERAPIST: How do you feel toward the part who protects Irene?

MAGGIE: (*Sighs.*) She thinks being Mom's slave will save us.

[*This slave is the parentified part.*]

THERAPIST: Has that been working?

MAGGIE: She thinks so.

THERAPIST: What works?

MAGGIE: (*Shrugs.*) Well, she's still alive and so am I!

THERAPIST: Does this part know who you are, Maggie?

MAGGIE: Me? She doesn't trust me.

THERAPIST: Why not?

MAGGIE: Because she thinks I want to, you know, erase the hard drive or something.

In this interchange, we hear that the parentified part did her best to buffer Maggie's internal system from Irene while also protecting Irene. Maggie's last comment, that the parentified part didn't want to know her, suggests that the parentified part was aware of Maggie's Self but wasn't ready to meet her.

● Maggie's Parentified Part Can't Do Enough

Here Maggie reported that her parentified part was accusing a promiscuous firefighter part of not doing enough for Irene, just as Irene would do.

MAGGIE: I give up! Nothing changes. Therapy isn't going to work on me.

THERAPIST: What doesn't change?

MAGGIE: I hear the same thing all the time!

THERAPIST: In your head? (*Maggie nods.*) What is it?

MAGGIE: Your mother drinks because of you. You're a bad daughter. You're selfish. You're sickening. All you want to do is get high and have sex. If you stayed home and took better care of Irene, she wouldn't hook up with a lowlife like Craig.

THERAPIST: Who does this critical part think you are?

MAGGIE: The one who picks up guys.

THERAPIST: And she's the one who takes care of Irene?

MAGGIE: Yeah.

THERAPIST: That's a big job. Wouldn't she like your help? I mean you, not the one who picks up guys.

● Maggie's Parentified Part Doesn't Trust Maggie's Self

In this conversation, I asked about college applications and found that Maggie was not following through with her plan to apply to colleges because the parentified part feared leaving Irene alone.

THERAPIST: Did you talk with your guidance counselor last week?

MAGGIE: Ah, no. Had to cancel.

THERAPIST: What's going on?

MAGGIE: (*Looks down.*) Hmm. I don't know about the college thing. All that debt and stuff. Maybe it's not me.

THERAPIST: What are you hearing inside?

MAGGIE: (*Looks up.*) One part is saying I can't leave Irene by herself. She'll get in trouble and I'll have to come home to take care of it, so I'll fail my classes anyway, have all that school debt, and end up working at McDonald's. I might as well go straight to McDonald's. I guess I'll just stay around here and find roommates.

THERAPIST: I thought you were applying to community colleges in this state?

MAGGIE: Well, I was looking at Texas or California or something.

THERAPIST: You have a part who wants to go far away, and another part who wants to stay nearby. We can talk about geography and school tuition, but first let's talk with the part who says you have to take care of Irene. Can you see that one?

MAGGIE: Yes.

THERAPIST: What does it look like?

MAGGIE: She's a giant octopus with something in every hand. A sponge, a spatula, a pad of paper, a pen. Like that.

THERAPIST: Who does she think you are?

MAGGIE: The little girl Irene steps on.

THERAPIST: What does she say to you?

MAGGIE: Don't worry. I've got this.

THERAPIST: She doesn't see you, the 17-year-old Maggie?

MAGGIE: No, she doesn't.

THERAPIST: Would she like to see you?

MAGGIE: She says, Why would I want to see you?

THERAPIST: What do you say? (*Maggie shrugs helplessly.*) Ask that part to relax for a moment. (*Maggie nods.*) What do you say?

MAGGIE: Maybe I could help.

THERAPIST: How does she respond?

MAGGIE: Okay. She sees me now. She says let's be sure not to aggravate Irene.

THERAPIST: That's her job?

MAGGIE: No. Her job is much bigger than that. She wants the little girl not to aggravate Irene.

THERAPIST: She thinks you're the little girl?

MAGGIE: No. She wants me to take care of the little girl so she can do her job.

THERAPIST: If you take care of the little girl, does she still need to do her job?

MAGGIE: (*Smiles.*) She thinks you're stupid.

THERAPIST: Who does she think you are?

MAGGIE: The babysitter.

The octopus part speaks of Irene as if she's a difficult child. It views her as a dependent and prioritizes her needs. As these snippets of Maggie's therapy illustrate, growing up doesn't stop parentified parts from fearing and feeling responsible for a dysfunctional caretaker. A parentified part needs attention first because it will interfere with exiles unburdening. Maggie was still young, just a teenager. The next example illustrates how enduring parentification can be.

● **Signey's Life Sentence: Parenting the Caretaker (and Everyone Else)**

Exiles who empathize and protectors who parent caretakers can remain bonded to that job throughout life. In therapy this phenomenon calls for patience, validation, and challenge. The following session with Signey, a cisgender, Swedish American lesbian in her 60s, occurred more than a year into therapy and illustrates one way of inquiring into the feelings of a parentified part. Signey remembered her father as largely absent (at work) while her stay-at-home mother, who had been adopted at the age of 3 and then profoundly neglected, devoted herself to her church and could not relate to children. When Signey was 12, her father was killed in a car accident. When she was 16, her mother sold their house and disappeared.

After that Signey took care of herself and anyone else in her orbit, including, eventually, her mother, who returned penniless. Signey's parentified part, who was chronically blended, didn't allow feelings. Whenever I asked Signey how she felt toward a part, she felt nothing. Even when she was weeping, she didn't register feelings. At the same time, she had palpable compassion for animals and children, and she understood (with tears but no feelings) that she had some desperately sad, lonely young parts. Her mother had been dead for many years by the time of this session, yet the idea of freedom from responsibility was still profoundly disorienting for her parentified part.

THERAPIST: You have a part who wants to protect your ex-girlfriend, your mother, your younger brother. It's altruistic and generous. It used to insist on spending holidays with your mother and brother, and it has insisted, over the objections of other parts, on spending holidays with your brother since his wife left him. What would happen if it stopped looking out for your brother?

SIGNEY: He would see how little interest I have in his life. He's clueless. He would have to see how small his life is.

THERAPIST: And then what would happen?

SIGNEY: He'd suffer.

THERAPIST: For your parts, what would be the worst thing about him suffering?

SIGNEY: I would be responsible.

THERAPIST: And what if you stopped being responsible?

SIGNEY: The headache is back.

THERAPIST: What does the headache want you to know?

SIGNEY: I have this impossible math part, you know: 2 plus 2 equals 5. But you're saying it equals 4.

THERAPIST: And what's the concern about that?

SIGNEY: It's like an earthquake. It would change the foundations of who I am. The building would fall down.

THERAPIST: Your parts built some rigid constraints to help you survive, but your body and mind are infinitely more flexible than a building.

SIGNEY: What would happen if I let my brother feel his feelings?

THERAPIST: What would happen?

SIGNEY: Why shouldn't he know how small his life is?

THERAPIST: Yeah, why?

SIGNEY: I feel responsible for his feelings.

THERAPIST: What would happen if you didn't take responsibility for his feelings?

SIGNEY: (*Tears.*) I know you're saying something true. I'm someone who faces the truth. But I don't know what to do with this. It's big.

Although this discussion merely hints at why this part would be alarmed to give up oppressive responsibilities, it does illustrate the foundational quality of a trauma bond for the protector who takes up the cause. The more dangerous or dependent the caretaker (or any proxy for the caretaker, such as an adult partner) is, the more likely it is that some part of the child, a part who is too young for responsibility but too smart to tolerate the consequences of declining it, will step into the parent role and insist on taking responsibility.

● Signey's Proxy Exile

Continuing with Signey's story, here is a session that occurred in short succession with the preceding one. Here Signey talks about her ex-girlfriend, Octavia.

SIGNEY: I'm reading books about childhood neglect, and they describe my childhood exactly. I want Octavia to read them. I think about knocking on her door all the time. I want her to know what I'm learning. This was her childhood, too. I think reading this could help her. But she doesn't want to hear from me. Why can't I let it go?

THERAPIST: How do you feel toward the part who doesn't let it go?

SIGNEY: I don't understand.

THERAPIST: Is it okay to be curious?

SIGNEY: The part seems anxious.

THERAPIST: Would it be willing to separate from you?

SIGNEY: Well, it just moved behind me when you said that.

THERAPIST: How do you feel toward it now?

SIGNEY: I'm curious.

THERAPIST: What does it want you to know?

SIGNEY: This must be the way the 2-year-old felt when she tried to connect with her mother and failed. (*Tearful.*) No one should have to suffer this way.

THERAPIST: Octavia puts up a wall—like your mother.

SIGNEY: Yes.

THERAPIST: But you know Octavia has parts behind this wall who feel hurt just like your 2-year-old. (*Signey nods.*) And you have a part who wants to help Octavia? (*She nods.*) Would it let you help your 2-year-old? (*Signey shakes her head no.*) What does it say about that?

SIGNEY: She tried everything.

THERAPIST: Who?

SIGNEY: The 2-year-old.

THERAPIST: She tried everything but nothing worked? What does this part do for the 2-year-old?

SIGNEY: It tells her to quit.

THERAPIST: It doesn't want her to feel hopeful, but it does want you to help Octavia's neglected young parts?

SIGNEY: It believes Octavia can be helped.

THERAPIST: And you can't be? (*Signey nods.*) Let's see if I'm understanding. This part doesn't want you to help the 2-year-old because since her mother isn't going to change she can't be helped? (*Signey nods.*) Does it mistake you for her mother?

SIGNEY: I don't know. It just wants me to help Octavia.

[*The part goes back to talking about Octavia.*]

THERAPIST: It wants you to help Octavia.

[*I follow suit.*]

SIGNEY: By the time I ended that relationship neither one of us could speak. We couldn't help each other. We were both neglected as children, and we both learned not to feel. I finally have hope that I'll get out of this. And this part really, really wants me to help Octavia, too. I don't know why it's so important.

Signey's 2-year-old part is stuck in a seminal moment when she tried to connect with her mother and got rejected. The part who takes care of others is not ready for her to help the 2-year-old. Rather, it wants to help her ex-girlfriend, with whom the 2-year-old empathizes and identifies. While this is not our ultimate destination, it is still a step in the direction of her exile. Notably, although Signey isn't afraid, ashamed, sad, or mad, she does feel guilt toward her mother, brother, and ex-girlfriend. That is, she only registers the principal feeling of her parentified protector and, vaguely, the emotional pain that her exiles feel when empathizing with Octavia's exiles. Nonetheless, Signey does have compassion for Octavia. Equally, she has compassion for little kids she sees on the street, and, occasionally, for her own young parts—so she feels hopeful.

● Gertrude and Jon: Differentiating to Resolve Maladaptive Guilt

This example, which features a family session between a caretaker and their adult child, who has a parentified part, illustrates empathy and guilt-based trauma bonding from two different perspectives. Jon, a 59-year-old, Norwegian American, cisgender, gay man, and Gertrude, his 76-year-old, cisgender, heterosexual mother, came to therapy to discuss his feelings about her new boyfriend. His biological father had committed suicide shortly after he was born, his first stepfather had been physically abusive with Gertrude, and his second stepfather had had bipolar disorder and had also committed suicide. Although Gertrude insisted that her new boyfriend, Al, was a kind man, Jon was unwilling to meet or socialize with him. When Gertrude asked for a few family therapy sessions to sort this out, Jon reluctantly agreed. Gertrude, who was in IFS therapy individually, chose an IFS therapist. This first session highlighted their trauma bonding history and the role empathy and identification were playing in their current impasse. We begin in the middle of the session, after I've guided them to speak for rather than from their parts.

JON: I don't want to be here.

THERAPIST: You have a part—

JON: I have parts who don't want to be here.

THERAPIST: (*To Gertrude.*) Are you open to hearing from those parts?

GERTRUDE: That's why I'm here.

THERAPIST: Okay, Jon. I'll help you speak for those parts, right? (*Jon nods.*)

But first, let's all go inside. We can ask our parts to relax and you can ask yours to let you speak for them. (*Everyone closes their eyes for a few moments.*) Ready? Jon, who wants to be spoken for first?

JON: I have an angry part. (*Hesitates for several beats, not making eye contact, then looks at Gertrude.*) Honestly, I don't know why he's so damn angry.

THERAPIST: Thanks. Before you continue, let me check with Gertrude. (*To Gertrude.*) When Jon says he has an angry part, what do you notice?

GERTRUDE: I know it, of course. But my heart sinks. I have many parts who feel sad when Jon does this.

THERAPIST: Does this?

GERTRUDE: I know why he's angry. He gets mad when I start a relationship. I know things haven't gone well in the past, and he has reason not to trust my judgment. I've made bad choices. But I was hoping he'd be willing to meet Al and decide for himself.

THERAPIST: What does your sad part need from you so you can listen to Jon?

GERTRUDE: No. I'm listening. It's okay.

THERAPIST: (*To Jon.*) Can you see your angry part? (Jon nods.) How old is he?

JON: About thirteen.

THERAPIST: How do you feel toward him?

JON: I like him.

THERAPIST: How does he respond?

JON: He's frustrated with me. And I'm hesitant to report his words about Gertrude.

GERTRUDE: It's okay.

JON: He says you're a self-involved ditz. (*Glances at Gertrude; she nods encouragingly.*)

THERAPIST: What does he want you and Gertrude to know?

JON: (*A few beats.*) When you . . . when this part of you gets all sparkly because some man pays attention, he feels dread. You leave him alone with our losses, pain, and outrage.

THERAPIST: What does he feel when Gertrude leaves him alone?

JON: Abandoned.

THERAPIST: I'm going to check in with Gertrude, okay? (*Jon nods.*) What do you notice inside right now?

GERTRUDE: I never wanted to burden Jon. I guess that's a part. How ironic!

I thought I was taking care of him by marrying again. I had a part who kept telling me I had to get myself off his hands, because he was such a responsible child, and I wanted him to have his own life as he grew up.

We met for several months after this initial session, allowing them to hear more from their parts and giving Gertrude time to apologize. Jon had parts who empathized and identified with his mother's vulnerable parts, and he had a parentified young part who felt responsible for her. This combination of *I am you* and *I am responsible for you* contributed to him vacillating between treating her like a twin and like a misbehaving ward. Their intimacy was intense, as were Jon's efforts to protect her, with the parentified boy alternately trying to control her and cutting her off for long periods of time. In therapy, Gertrude identified and helped her exiled parts, who had recruited Jon to take care of her, and also the protector who tried to counter this by finding an adult man to take care of her; but she had chosen men who were overly attentive and then controlling and rageful. Meanwhile, Jon helped his parentified 13-year-old let go of feeling responsible for her.

Trauma Bonding and the Higher Self

As we see with Maggie, Signey, and Jon, parentified parts can act like frantic, if annoyed, parents who are willing to make significant personal sacrifices to avoid what they fear will be a bad outcome for the nominal caretaker. They believe that the status quo is safest and that unilateral liberation from a dependent caretaker would be cruel and perhaps dangerous. They're well behaved and overly responsible. Challenged grown-ups like and encourage them, and we ignore them in therapy at our peril.

If we can include the client's nominal caretaker(s) in therapy sessions— if they're willing to come and safe enough to include—then family sessions are preferable, especially for teens and young adults, but even for older adults. That said, caretakers may be unwilling, geographically distant, dead, or otherwise largely irrelevant to the client's life today. If logic hasn't released the parentified part from its job under those circumstances, attention and help are in order. Parentified parts need help—but of a particular kind. They're worn-out children whose grim determination aims to keep a meager version of hope alive. If I'm loyal, I can hope to save you; I can hope that we'll reconcile and you'll love me. They hope for redemption, fear future guilt, and focus on the caretaker's welfare with a single-minded concern that ultimately puts them at odds with the needs of the internal system they once aimed to protect. This kind of conflict is best addressed, I find, with compassion for everyone involved: for the attached young exiles who want to save their caretaker's exiles, for the angry parts who want justice, and for the parentified part who is caught in the middle and longs for the caretaker to behave. And also, compassion for the caretaker.

When a nominal caretaker looks to their offspring for parenting, they are caught in an intergenerational pattern of role reversal. In each generation, the child is inducted into feeling responsible for the caretaker, who probably also took care of their nominal caretaker and has exiled parts who were emotionally (and often literally) deprived. In this way, no generation gets sufficient attention, safety, nurture, or love. This deprivation is continually bequeathed to another chosen child (perhaps the oldest, the only, or the most capable) until some rebellious offspring finds a way to intervene on their own behalf—as we hope our clients are doing in therapy. Before then, the parentified child is doomed to an ongoing battle between parts who long for nourishment and parts who sacrifice personal needs in service of survival. In IFS we say the parentified child, a protector, inherited the job of self-sacrifice.

Naturally, parentified parts long for transgressing caretakers to acknowledge the harm they've done, which makes it harder for them to resolve their trauma bond by letting them go. This came home to me with particular clarity as I was learning to do legacy unburdenings (Sinko, 2017), which are a ceremonial way for ancestors to join the client in letting go of inherited burdens. I had studied up and was following advice, but I kept running into the same obstacles, including (1) one part of the client objecting fiercely to the idea of including the caretaker, whereas another part, loyal and equally intense, was refusing to leave the past without having helped the caretaker; (2) the caretaker showing up as they did in life—aggressive, threatening, and misbehaving, or refusing to participate; and (3) a part of the client who wanted to include some ancestors but exclude others, which would leave unfinished business.

Understandable as these demands and objections were, they kept my clients from resolving the intergenerational conflict that consumed so much of their mental and emotional time. With low expectations and a sense of defeat, I kept trying. My clients needed ancestral accountability. How to get it? Finally, during the following session, I thought of doing what we always do in IFS (calling on the Self). Here's what happened.

Renata and Her Father: Accessing the Self in Everyone

Renata, a 40-year-old, cisgender, single, Norwegian American woman, grew up with an angry mother who was not shy about declaring that she had married down. Renata's mother had little interest in parenting and would often put a large bowl of popcorn out for her three children at mealtimes and then lie on the couch reading. She tolerated no complaints, no sibling rivalry, no demands, and no emotional needs. She criticized Renata in front of her peers and other parents at school events and ignored her at home. In turn, Renata clung to her older sister, Klara, and was mean to her younger brother, Andre, about which she felt exceedingly guilty later in life.

Renata's father, a plumber, was out of the house much of the time. In addition to having a unionized day job, he worked nights and weekends. But when he was at home, he smoldered. Raging, criticizing, threatening, demeaning, he duplicated the behavior of his own father, who he despised. Renata had parts who feared he would kill her, were devastated by his obvious distress, and wondered whether or not to say hello to him in the morning. If she did say hello, he seemed to feel she was intruding (Was she hurting him? Was it too painful for him?). If she didn't say hello, he seemed insulted and scowled more deeply (Was he suffering? Would he attack her?).

She had a team of parts who tried to please both parents. They also tried shutting up, avoiding people altogether, and frowning. She had parts who longed for attention. She had a part who soothed herself by rocking in the rocking chair in Klara's empty bedroom, for Klara had fled home as soon as she could, leaving 8-year-old Renata and 5-year-old Andre to face their parents alone. In this session, which occurred more than a year into therapy, Renata had her first opportunity to help an exile—the one who had spent hours rocking herself—to unburden. But another part interrupted.

RENATA: No. It's not possible.

THERAPIST: This part can't unburden her feeling of worthlessness?

RENATA: What about him?

THERAPIST: Who?

RENATA: My father.

THERAPIST: What do you hear about your father?

RENATA: My mother mauled him and then left. I can't leave him.

THERAPIST: What would happen if you left him?

RENATA: I can't.

[*Her father, by the way, had died of cancer at least 10 years prior to this session.*]

THERAPIST: Is this one part or more?

RENATA: Lots of parts. We can't leave him.

THERAPIST: Shall we help him, then? (*Renata nods.*) Can you see him now? (*Renata nods.*) Does he see you? (*She shakes her head no.*) Ask if he would like to see you and get help.

[*This was my ah-ha! moment.*]

RENATA: Yes.

THERAPIST: Okay. Let's start by calling in his higher Self. Let me know when it's there. (*Renata nods.*) What needs to happen now?

RENATA: He wants to apologize.

THERAPIST: Is that okay with you? (*Renata nods and sits silently with her eyes closed; after a couple of minutes, she opens her eyes.*)

RENATA: He's sorry.

THERAPIST: If you want to say something to him, his higher Self can help him listen and understand.

RENATA: I feel sad that we went through this. He's nodding. He can see perfectly now. (*Pauses.*) Where will he go?

THERAPIST: He can go with his higher Self when you're ready.

RENATA: She wants to burn the worthless feeling. He has it, too. Can he put his in the fire?

THERAPIST: What do you say?

RENATA: Yes! And he wants to invite his father and his father's father with their higher Selves. It goes back and back.

THERAPIST: What needs to happen?

RENATA: Everyone who's ready can put their burdens in the fire.

THERAPIST: And if they're not ready?

RENATA: They can go with their higher Selves for help.

This session shows Renata's parentified part turning responsibility for her father over to his Self so the two of them, along with his ancestors, can release the burdens he visited on her. Once we included her father's higher Self, Renata's parentified part was quick to hand control of the session to her Self, as we see in her confident handling of the intergenerational unburdening that followed. Witnessing how well this worked with Renata, I tried it with a number of other clients and concluded that it generally works well. To my surprise, no one has yet questioned the idea that their caretaker had (or has) a higher Self. But I do have one caveat. A client who was terrorized by a sadistic caretaker may not be ready for any kind of contact. In this case, don't push or insist. The client knows best.

EXERCISE

Letting Go of Inherited Burdens and Including the Ancestor's Higher Self

You can do this exercise with a client or with your own parts. If you notice a protector who won't unblend, or who seems allergic to your Self rather than relieved at your presence, ask the part if it has a trauma bond with a caretaker. This bond may be based on identification and shame or responsibility and guilt—or both. If there is a trauma bond, find the part (or parts) who are involved and follow this exercise. Take notes.

1. Start by turning your attention inside and asking the part who doesn't trust the client's Self who it protects.

2. If it names a caretaker or some other relative, ask what would happen if it didn't protect this person.

3. If the part names a fear that was relevant in the past but is no longer relevant, let it know that you are grown up now and ask if it would like a tour of your present life.

4. If not, ask why.

5. If yes, show it around your present and see if it would like to come and live with you—or go someplace else out of the past.

6. If yes, ask if it is ready to release its caretaking bond along with any other inherited burdens, and then ask if it would like to include the higher Self of ancestors in the unburdening process.

Conclusion

Most manager parts fear the client being exposed as unlovable, but parentified managers cling to burdensome bonds from fear of what will happen if the client isn't loving enough. Tasked with big responsibilities early in life and fearing inner criticism in perpetuity should they give up on the impossible task of rescuing the caretaker from their fears or demons, parentified managers are in a permanent pickle. They feel guilty now and fear feeling guilty in the future. Trauma bonding—loyalty, responsibility, unexpressed anger, maladaptive guilt, and an unmet longing for repair—can thwart the system's ability to reach consensus, let go of personal burdens, and leave the past. But with patience, dogged attention to the client's trauma bonds, and the help of a caretaker's higher Self, we can help parentified parts let go.

SECTION II

Treatment

In the first section of this book, I employed numerous scenes from therapy to illustrate various assertions. Whether you agree with those assertions or not, I hope they and the illustrations that go with them captured your attention and will enrich your personal and professional explorations in the future. We turn now to a more orderly presentation of my treatment recommendations for readers who are using IFS or want to give it a try.

THE FIRST PORTION OF THERAPY

CHAPTER 8

Set the Stage

In this and the next two chapters (9 and 10), I focus on the first portion of therapy, in which protectors call the shots. In Chapter 11, I present the second portion of therapy, when exiles get free rein. Divided into these two portions, the basic procedure of IFS is linear and straightforward. First, we ask protectors to unblend; if they decline, we ask why; then we offer to help with their concerns. Eventually, they permit us to help exiled parts, and we move to the second portion of therapy, witnessing and unburdening exiles. The art of practicing IFS begins when progress stops being linear. Say, for example, protectors aren't willing to unblend and won't say why. What to do then? In this chapter, I illustrate some strategies for maintaining flow as obstacles arise in the therapy hour. We can:

- Pose hypotheticals to anxious, naysayer protectors.
- Use the U-turn to redirect protector projections and promote internal relationships.
- Challenge protectors to separate and meet the Self—the obstacle is willingness, not ability. If they're not willing, our job is to find out why and address their concerns.
- Tell protectors that the Self can help injured young parts because (1) the Self is not a part; (2) exiles aren't bad (a bad thing happened to them); and (3) the past may not change, but exiles can rewrite their story and leave the past.

Regardless of whether you are in the first portion, helping protectors, or the second, witnessing exiles, you will be well served in the therapist role if you check on your parts and gauge your Self-energy. How spacious—or crowded—are your mind and body? You might feel relaxed and expansive, or you might notice a sense of aversion or a feeling of dread and restriction inside. If you notice any negative feeling or sensation, pause and inquire. Is one of your parts reacting to this client? What does it want you to know? Does it need your help? If so, this marks a good spot for exploration in your system. Set an intention to return and help the distressed part, then ask it (and all other parts) to let you take the lead for the next hour. To practice going inside and getting to know your protectors, follow the steps in the box below. If you have smooth sailing, find an exile and set the intention to help it. If your protectors don't cooperate, this chapter will show you how to keep a session in flow. Read it and try again.

The Standard Procedure for the First Portion of IFS Therapy

Follow the procedure described here with your own protective parts. This is the first portion of IFS therapy. Practicing with your system will help you recognize clues to shaming, shamefulness, and guilt and will teach you how to navigate common choice points.

- Start with a target part—be sure it's a protector.
  - To find out if the part is a protector, just ask if it protects anyone. If it says *no*, it's an exile. Ask it to wait, and promise to return when you can.
  - If the part refuses to answer or says *yes*, then it is a protector.
  - In any case, find a protector to interview.
- Once you have a protector in mind, describe it.
- How do you feel toward it? Help any reactive protectors who show up to relax back.
- When you feel something in the ballpark of curiosity, kindness, or compassion toward the target part, ask it some questions:
  - What does it do for you, who does it protect, who does it disagree with, and what would happen if it stopped doing its job?
- If it fears the behavior of another protector, offer to help with that conflict.
- If it names a vulnerability, offer to help that exile.

Getting in the Middle of a Protector Polarity without Taking a Side

To intervene in a protector polarity, convene a meeting of both parts (or teams of parts) with your Self.

- Make sure they see you, and also make sure that you are at the table with them (e.g., not floating above).

- Describe the parts at the table.
- Ask them who needs attention first, and then ask that part these questions:
  - What do you do for me?
  - Who do you protect?
  - Who do you disagree with?
  - And what would happen if you stopped doing this job?
- Then do the same with a part on the other side of the table.
- Finally, ask them all to notice that the part they protect, whether it's the same part or a different one, is hurt and tell them you could take care of the hurt part if they were willing.
- Stay with them until they agree.

Once protectors agree, you're ready to move into the second portion of therapy. If you want to keep going, skip up to Chapter 11, where the action shifts from protectors to exiles. Otherwise, thank the protectors, make a note, and set an intention to help this exile later on.

Listen for Shaming, Shamefulness, and Guilt from the Beginning of Therapy

As the client speaks, whether in the first session or those that follow, listen for shaming. Does the client shame themselves? Do they shame others? Or do they feel guilty toward someone else? If they feel guilty, is their guilt adaptive or maladaptive? And, finally, do they feel wronged by someone else? Here are examples of all these options.

Shaming

The Client Shames Themself

Almira is 18 years old. She starts therapy sessions by talking about her weight: *Look how fat I am!* Or *How do I look? I've been running and I lost 5 pounds. Can you tell?* She speaks critically of herself and invites the therapist to be either a nonprotecting bystander or an active judge. Here is how I might speak with a client who shames themself in therapy:

ALMIRA: Look how fat I am. Can you tell?

THERAPIST: You have a part who criticizes you in front of me and then invites me to comment. Let's think about my options here. What would it be like for you if I contradicted this critic?

ALMIRA: (*Considers.*) I'd think you're a phony and you won't tell the truth.

THERAPIST: Anything else?

ALMIRA: I'd think you're trying to be nice, but it's pointless.

THERAPIST: More? (*Almira shakes her head.*) And what would you feel?

ALMIRA: Sad.

THERAPIST: Okay. Let's think about some other options. If I said nothing, what would you hear inside?

ALMIRA: *She thinks you're disgusting. Why do you go fishing for reassurance when you know it's true?*

THERAPIST: Anything else?

ALMIRA: *At least this therapist is honest.*

THERAPIST: And anything else?

ALMIRA: Yes. Two things. *You could kill yourself now.* And, *Maybe you should try a new therapist.*

THERAPIST: And what would you feel?

ALMIRA: (*Considers.*) Confused.

THERAPIST: Okay. Other options. Let's see. What if I agreed?

ALMIRA: I'd feel betrayed, get really mad, and I wouldn't want to come next week. (*A pause.*) And I'd probably go on a really strict diet.

THERAPIST: Lots of parts.

ALMIRA: Yeah.

THERAPIST: How do you feel toward the part who asks me that question?

ALMIRA: I pity it. It's just copying my sister and other girls.

THERAPIST: It wants something for you. What does it want?

ALMIRA: Rescue.

THERAPIST: From?

ALMIRA: Criticizing myself, I guess.

THERAPIST: Does it work?

ALMIRA: No.

THERAPIST: We could talk to the critic directly, though. Want to do that?

ALMIRA: I guess we better.

● The Client Shames Someone Else

Here is how I might speak with a client who shames others in therapy. Eric is 18 years old and often starts therapy sessions by speaking about other people critically. For example, he might say, *There's this imbecile in my calculus class . . .* Like Almira, Eric is inviting the therapist to be a nonprotecting bystander or a proxy judge.

ERIC'S CRITIC: There's this imbecile in my calculus class who really bugs me. He shouldn't be there. He holds everyone back.

THERAPIST: How do you feel toward the part who calls your classmate an imbecile?

ERIC'S CRITIC: It's observant.

[*From this snarky answer, I conclude that the critical part is blended.*]

THERAPIST: How about I talk with it and you listen? (*Eric nods.*) In what way does this kid bug you?

ERIC'S CRITIC: He's stupid.

THERAPIST: You mean, he struggles with the concepts of calculus?

ERIC'S CRITIC: Okay, he struggles and the teacher explains.

THERAPIST: And what's the worst thing about that for you?

ERIC'S CRITIC: It's embarrassing.

THERAPIST: Because?

ERIC'S CRITIC: He's pitiful and weak.

THERAPIST: And what's worst about being pitiful and weak?

ERIC'S CRITIC: You'll be squashed like a bug.

THERAPIST: Who do you protect?

ERIC'S CRITIC: (*A long pause.*) You know.

THERAPIST: I can guess. Is it okay if I guess? (*Eric nods.*) You protect the little boy who got hurt by his angry brother and his distracted, temperamental dad. (*Eric nods.*) I've said Eric could help that boy.

ERIC'S CRITIC: Yeah, yeah.

THERAPIST: I don't want you to take my word for it. I want you to meet the Eric-who's-not-a-part and decide for yourself. Are you willing?

ERIC'S CRITIC: Okay. Maybe.

As these examples illustrate, if you hear shaming, it's an opportunity to get curious about the part who's doing the shaming. Whether a critic is shaming internally or externally, it is marking an important concern for the client, and we need to get curious about what it's doing. No doubt it has an effect on other parts and on the client's behavior. It's a good place to start.

● The Client Feels Shameful

The client talks of feeling shameful, either directly or indirectly. Here is how that might sound and what I might say. Gemma, who is 33 years old, avoids many interactions and opportunities.

GEMMA: I got invited to a birthday party by a couple I don't know very well.

THERAPIST: Are you going?

GEMMA: It was last weekend. I didn't go. (*Pause.*) I can't go to parties. I disapparate and become, you know, like atoms, not a body or a person. It takes days to recover.

[*To* disapparate, *a concept the Harry Potter generation understands, is to* "*magically disappear.*"]

THERAPIST: Who disapparates?

GEMMA: I don't know.

THERAPIST: Ask.

GEMMA: A scared part.

THERAPIST: What is it scared of?

GEMMA: People.

THERAPIST: What is scary about people?

GEMMA: They see you.

THERAPIST: And then?

GEMMA: You're revealed.

THERAPIST: And then?

GEMMA: You feel like you have to jump out of your skin to escape.

THERAPIST: Because.

GEMMA: They've seen you.

THERAPIST: And what's the worst thing about being seen?

GEMMA: They know how worthless and bad and disgusting you are.

THERAPIST: You have a part who feels that way. When everyone is ready, we can help that part. Would that be good? (*Gemma nods.*) Ask if anyone objects to you helping the part who feels worthless, bad, and disgusting.

Gemma names a part who feels shameful. Unlike talking with a shaming manager, we have to be cautious about pursuing a part like this, who is likely an exile. Notice that I say we can help the part, but I also say we have to get permission.

Guilt

If you don't hear shaming, you may hear guilt. This, also, is a communication about a problem that needs to be solved. Is the client expressing guilt directly or indirectly? Is their guilt adaptive or maladaptive? Here are examples.

● The Client Feels Guilty about Transgressing

In the first session, Vera said she felt guilty about her son's suicide. She had never known, she said, how to respond to his depression. She recounted the ways in which she had invalidated, resented, and abandoned him since he first got depressed in early adolescence when she divorced his father, who was chronically depressed and unemployed. Although some features of her story may have been exaggerated, I had the impression that her son's death had jolted the parts she was describing into unblending and that she was seeing her behavior from a new angle. At the same time, her parts were seeing her son (whom they had confused with her ex-husband) from a new angle. As a result, she was feeling deep remorse, which seemed adaptive to me. The shaming condemnations of her inner critics, however, were maladaptive and would interfere with her ability to feel compassion for the parts who had made this mistake.

● The Client Acts As If They Feel Guilty, Even Though They Have Not Transgressed against Anyone

Malcolm ended a relationship after repeated attempts to help his girlfriend stop drinking. She later developed cirrhosis of the liver and died awaiting a transplant. In therapy, he said he regretted ending the relationship. On inquiry, however, it became clear that he did not regret ending the relationship; he had parts who felt guilty about not rescuing her. They told him that he could have succeeded if he had tried harder. This guilt, expressed indirectly (*I wish I hadn't ended the relationship*), was maladaptive.

● The Client Feels Wounded

The client believes they were wronged and expresses a sense of injury. River broke up with their partner, Sam, and then River's best friend got into a romantic relationship with Sam. River felt betrayed by their best friend and by Sam. Distracting from exiled feelings of worthlessness and despair, River's managers vowed never to be in a relationship again. It told River not to trust people and not to get into another intimate relationship. Meanwhile, River's firefighters were cooking up fantasies of revenge. All this got in the way of River helping their sad exile who was feeling unlovable. Take note when you hear a client's parts shaming, feeling shameful, feeling guilty, or feeling wronged. It's likely to be a theme in their experience more broadly and to mark a trail that will lead back to injuring experiences earlier in life.

In short, expressions of shamefulness, guilt, paranoia, revenge, or hurt are all an opportunity to track down injured, exiled parts.

Talking about Parts

Whether you're meeting with a client for the first time or you're in the middle of treatment, talk about parts. Listen to your client and translate what they say into parts language. Here are some ways of ensuring that you will be talking about parts in therapy.

Translate the Client's Words to Parts Language

TOM'S WORRIED MANAGER: I planned to do all this work around the house over the weekend, but I didn't do any of it! I did other stuff, not what I need to get done. This happens all the time. What's wrong with me?

THERAPIST: You have a part who planned to do all this work around the house over the weekend but didn't do it because another part got in the driver's seat and did other stuff. You also have a part who notices this happening all the time and wonders if something is wrong with you. Is that right?

Once you've tagged all the parts the client names, you can ask who needs attention first.

Listen to Stories, but Talk Parts

Sometimes a client insists on *telling a story* or giving you an *update* before—or instead of—noticing their parts. You, however, can listen for parts and respond by talking about them. Here is an example.

VIOLA'S REPORTING MANAGER: I just need to talk about my week. It was so stressful! My roommate threw up all over the living room rug Saturday night because they drink too much. My cat escaped because my roommate's boyfriend left the door open, and I had to go into that creepy basement to find him. And I got a B-minus on my final English paper! I really thought it was an A, you know? I worked really hard. This professor is such a flint ass. And I don't want to go home for Christmas.

THERAPIST: No?

VIOLA'S REPORTING MANAGER: Why go home to be cold and hungry?

THERAPIST: You said a lot just now, Viola. Your roommate and their boyfriend are difficult. You didn't get the response you expected from your English professor. And you expect to be deprived when you go home. What do you feel right now?

VIOLA'S REPORTING MANAGER: Miserable.

THERAPIST: Right. You have parts who find all that very challenging. Would they like your help?

If a Client Objects to Talking about Parts, You Can Use Their Language

MEENA'S CONCERNED MANAGER: I need therapy because I'm too anxious.

THERAPIST: You have an anxious part.

MEENA'S CONCERNED MANAGER: I don't know what you mean by *part*. Can we just talk regular?

THERAPIST: Sure. Tell me about your anxiety.

MEENA'S CONCERNED MANAGER: I've always been anxious. I was an anxious little girl. My two older brothers scared me, and I'm always afraid of failing.

THERAPIST: How do you feel toward this anxiety, Meena?

MEENA'S CONCERNED MANAGER: I don't like it.

THERAPIST: Understandable. Could we be curious about the anxiety even though it's been such a challenge?

MEENA'S CONCERNED MANAGER: Oh. I guess so. Sometimes I think if I just don't pay attention, it will go away.

THERAPIST: Does that work?

MEENA'S CONCERNED MANAGER: No.

THERAPIST: Let's see if we can notice it safely. Where do you find it?

MEENA: In my stomach.

THERAPIST: Knowing that it feels anxious about something, could you feel some kindness toward it?

MEENA: I guess so.

THERAPIST: What color do you associate with kindness?

MEENA: Hmmm. Greeny-blue.

THERAPIST: Put some greeny-blue light in the palm of your hand and bring it to your stomach. (*Meena does this.*) Now ask the anxiety not to overwhelm you in exchange for you paying attention.

MEENA: Okay.

THERAPIST: How's that?

MEENA: Better.

THERAPIST: Is it okay to hear from the anxiety now? (*Meena nods.*) What does it want you to know?

You Can Ask Them to Try Your Language

MEENA'S CONCERNED MANAGER: I wake up in the night and can't get back to sleep.

THERAPIST: What happens when you wake up?

MEENA'S CONCERNED MANAGER: I think about all the mistakes I've made in my life, and I can't stop.

THERAPIST: So, some part of you wakes you up and then shows or tells you about a lot of stuff from the past that you regret.

MEENA'S CONCERNED MANAGER: What do you mean *some part of you*?

THERAPIST: I mean our minds don't just go on one track at a time. In this case, one part of you—or maybe lots of parts—want to sleep, but another part shows you this stuff. We don't know why.

MEENA'S CONCERNED MANAGER: Well, I don't think of myself that way.

THERAPIST: Would you be willing to give it a try?

MEENA'S CONCERNED MANAGER: What's the point?

THERAPIST: It will give you a new way of thinking about—and relating to—yourself, which I promise will be interesting.

MEENA'S CONCERNED MANAGER: (*Shrugs.*) I don't know.

THERAPIST: Do you hear a concern about trying something new?

MEENA'S CONCERNED MANAGER: I'm not crazy, you know. I just can't sleep.

THERAPIST: We all have parts. It's normal.

MEENA'S CONCERNED MANAGER: But what if I hear things I don't want to hear?

THERAPIST: I think that is already happening. The idea would be to make it safe for you to hear anything that any part wants to tell you. We can do that. I'm betting that would help you sleep at night again.

MEENA'S CONCERNED MANAGER: How can you make it safe?

THERAPIST: Can I show you?

Or Try Making a Deal: You Say *Feelings*, I'll Say *Parts*

CALISTA'S WARY MANAGER: I don't know what you mean by *part*. Can't we just be regular?

THERAPIST: Are you open to a little experiment?

CALISTA'S WARY MANAGER: What?

THERAPIST: Well, talking about parts *is* regular for me. So how about you talk about your experience, and I'll tell you what I'm hearing in the language I normally use. That way, you can hear how I think about things and see if it appeals.

CALISTA's WARY MANAGER: Okay. Yeah, I want to know how you think.

THERAPIST: This meeting will help you decide if what I offer suits you.

CALISTA's WARY MANAGER: That's right. I am shopping around. My mom told me I should feel comfortable with a therapist.

THERAPIST: I agree. So, you tell me what you want from therapy in your words, and I'll tell you what I'm hearing in my words.

CALISTA's WARY MANAGER: Okay. I can do that.

Of course, finding language that works for all parties is crucial in any approach or modality of therapy. Language matters. When using the IFS frame, talking about parts and so forth, clients may initially find the language strange, exotic, or childish. Focusing on this will help the therapeutic alliance.

EXERCISE

Starting Therapy

In this exercise, practice starting a new therapy in your imagination. You can think back to a session with a new client. As you answer the following questions, take notes.

- Picture the client, remember their story, and ask yourself (as you will in subsequent sessions):
  - How much internal space do I have?
  - What feelings do I notice?
- If, for example, you have anxiety or dread about the upcoming meeting, ask why and listen. Your parts may have some guidance for you, or they may need your help.
  - This is an initial session. What does the client say? Do they shame themself or others as they tell their story?
  - Also listen for guilt. Does the client express guilt? If so, does it sound adaptive (they really did transgress) or maladaptive (they were pursuing normal developmental goals)?
  - Translate the client's story into parts language as they go along.
  - If the client objects to talking about parts, consider three options and choose one.
    - You can use their language.
    - You can ask them to try using your language.
    - Or you can make a deal that you will each use the language you prefer and then talk about it.

The Word *Work*

Do we need our clients to sign on for more work? Notice how you use the word *work* to signify the therapy process and remember that you're mostly talking with child parts. Try substituting some of the words below or find words you prefer. In any case, you can convey your meaning more precisely than by using the single word *work* all the time. But one caveat: Managers, who are sure to have put themselves to work of necessity when they were young and will have been working too hard for too long, may show alarm when you invite them to stop working. At the same time, the idea of not working will intrigue them. We invite young managers to quit working so hard. We want to relieve them of grown-up responsibilities so they can play, explore, and learn as children ought. Here is a list of alternatives, by no means comprehensive.

- *Explore.*
- *Inquire.*
- *Help.*
- *Learn.*
- *Review.*
- *Experiment.*
- *Try.*

Seamus Is Working Too Hard

Here is an example of using the word **work** (bolded) to describe what protectors do but substituting the words **explore** and **inquire** (also **bolded**) when talking about the process of therapy.

SEAMUS: I'm coming to therapy to **work** on my depression.

THERAPIST: Okay. Let's **explore** your depression. Tell me about it.

SEAMUS: From where anyone else is sitting, I have a good life. How many actors can actually earn a living acting? I've had some great breaks. I'm incredibly lucky. Why don't I feel it?

THERAPIST: What do you notice instead?

SEAMUS: Just flat. No enthusiasm. The more I get what I want, the less I want to get out of bed. I do, of course, because I'm a good actor.

THERAPIST: Say more.

SEAMUS: I've always had this problem. I want something, I focus on it, I go for it fiercely. But if I succeed, I'm overtaken by this huge letdown.

THERAPIST: So, I'm hearing that some parts of you **work** really hard but don't enjoy success at the end of all that hard **work**. They can't celebrate for some reason. Is that right?

SEAMUS: Yes. Why?

THERAPIST: That's a great question. *Why can't I enjoy success?*

SEAMUS: So how would you **work** on this?

THERAPIST: I would help you **inquire** inside. You've described parts who **work** really hard, and parts who feel let down when you succeed and stop **working**. Right? (*Seamus nods.*) So, first I'd ask, *Who feels let down? The hardworking parts or some other part?*

SEAMUS: Another part.

THERAPIST: Does it feel disappointed when the **hardworking** parts don't have any more **work** to do? Or does the let-down part feel bad all along and you only notice it when you're not **working** hard?

SEAMUS: That one.

THERAPIST: So, the **hardworking** parts distract from a part who feels bad? (*Seamus nods.*) What if you could help it?

SEAMUS: That would be great.

The Word *Change*

Protectors need to hear a few things from you up front: (1) You're not trying to control or change them; (2) exiled parts also don't need to change; (3) you and the client honor their hard work, and you're here to offer them and the exiles they protect the resources of the client's Self so they don't have to keep working so hard in the future; and (4) they can experiment with new options without making any commitment. After all, being scientific means having a hypothesis and being willing to be proved wrong.

● ANDY Doesn't Need to Change

Here is an example of substituting other words for the word *change*.

ANDY'S FIREFIGHTER: I hate to tell you this, but I'm only here because my wife says she'll leave if I don't stop looking at pornography. I like it, so how am I supposed to stop? I stop, I start, I do it on the QT, but she's got this sixth sense and becomes a . . . you know, cop. It's ruining our marriage. But, honestly, I don't know if I can stop. I've been doing it since I was 12 years old. It's just an old habit.

THERAPIST: What do you like about it?

ANDY'S FIREFIGHTER: It's comforting. It calms me down when I feel bad.

THERAPIST: A part shows you pornography to comfort you when you feel bad. (*Andy nods.*) But your wife objects. (*Andy nods.*) If she didn't object, would you have any concerns?

ANDY'S FIREFIGHTER: Like what?

THERAPIST: I don't know.

ANDY: You mean, like, I'm not so interested in actual sex?

THERAPIST: Yeah, that kind of thing.

ANDY: I do feel kind of flat. So, I go back for more. And it is harder. . . . I hope I can speak frankly? It is harder to have an erection if I overuse.

THERAPIST: (*Nods.*) Is that how your wife can tell?

ANDY'S FIREFIGHTER: Probably. But I don't think I can change.

THERAPIST: So, here's the thing. I'm not interested in changing any of your parts. The part who shows you pornography has a good reason. It helps when you feel bad. I don't want us to try to change or control any part who's helping you. But I do want us to help the part who feels bad.

ANDY'S FIREFIGHTER: I don't think that part can be helped.

THERAPIST: Why?

ANDY'S FIREFIGHTER: Because that's who I am.

THERAPIST: Tell me, Andy, when you feel bad, what are you hearing inside?

ANDY: *You're an asshole.* Pardon my language, *You're a piece of shit.*

THERAPIST: No wonder you feel bad. (*Andy nods glumly.*) When you hear that, what do you believe about yourself?

ANDY: I'm a worthless piece of . . . you know, trash.

THERAPIST: Let me sum up. Okay? (*Andy nods.*) You have a part who feels worthless, another part who is harsh and calls you names—

ANDY: (*Interrupting.*) And sounds like my father.

THERAPIST: And sounds like your father. And another part who helps you survive that cruelty with pornography, which is soothing.

ANDY'S FIREFIGHTER: Yes.

THERAPIST: So, we don't want to stop the pornography part from helping you when you need help. But wouldn't it be great if you felt good and didn't need that help? Then the pornography part would be free to do something else—whatever it wanted. It could go back to being who it was meant to be before it had to save you from feeling worthless.

ANDY'S FIREFIGHTER: How am I supposed to feel good?

THERAPIST: I promise it's possible. We'd start by talking with your father's voice. Does it belong to you? I mean, is it one of your parts copying him?

ANDY: (*Considers.*) Yes.

THERAPIST: This part copies your father's voice and uses his energy?

ANDY: Yes. And he wants you to know he can't change.

THERAPIST: Okay. We're not going to ask him to change. You know why? Because he's a good guy. Like the pornography part, he's just trying to help. (*A pause while Andy considers.*) Can I ask him a question? (*Andy nods.*) What does he want for you?

ANDY'S MANAGER: He wants me to stop being such an—

THERAPIST: (*Interrupting.*) I know he's good at criticizing you. In fact, he's great at it. But we're asking him to take a break from doing that right now and tell you *why* he does it. What are his hopes for you?

ANDY'S MANAGER: That I'll be loved.

THERAPIST: See? There's nothing more important than what he wants for you. Do his tactics work?

ANDY'S MANAGER: Well . . . no. But I can't just look at pornography all day long!

THERAPIST: No, you can't. That solution doesn't work except in the very short run. But I can show you a better way if this critic and the pornography part are willing.

ANDY: The critic is afraid Mr. Porn will take over if he goes soft (*smiles bashfully*), so to speak.

THERAPIST: Okay. Ask Mr. Porn if he can agree to a truce.

ANDY: He says, *It's a two-way street, buddy.*

THERAPIST: That's right. They would both have to agree and follow through. But we'll start with an easy, quick truce. They could just lay down their arms here, when we're all together, where you can be the third party and keep them both honest. Remember, they aren't agreeing to anything permanent, just an experiment to see what's possible for the future. I promise they're going to like having you around.

ANDY: Okay. They agree.

Clarify the Client's Language

What Does *I Understand* Mean?

THERAPIST: How do you feel toward this part?

ROBERT: I understand.

THERAPIST: Tell it what you understand and ask if you have it right. Does it want you to know anything else?

What Does *I Feel Sad* Mean?

THERAPIST: How do you feel toward this part?

MARGOT: Sad.

THERAPIST: What kind of sad?

MARGOT: Sad for the part.

THERAPIST: Pity or concern?

MARGOT: Concern.

In Addition to Using Language with Care, Assess the Client's Sensory Experience

Ask the client if they're visual. If not, explore how they experience their parts. Maybe they sense, feel, or hear parts rather than seeing them. Either way, ask them to describe parts according to their experience and inquire about the age of each part as it comes up. Here are two examples.

● Frankie Experiences Their Parts Visually, Aurally, and Kinesthetically

THERAPIST: So, tell me, Frankie, how do you become aware of a part?

FRANKIE: Sometimes I see it. Sometimes I feel it. And sometimes I hear it speak or notice what it's doing.

THERAPIST: And how do you know what you feel is a part?

FRANKIE: At first, I don't. But if I pay attention and ask some questions, it becomes clear.

THERAPIST: What questions do you ask?

FRANKIE: I might ask a sensation or a feeling, *What do you want me to know?* If there's no answer, I ask, *Is this a part?*

THERAPIST: And if you get no answer in both cases?

FRANKIE: (*Shrugs.*) Yeah. With sensations I might go more toward, you know, this is just a body thing.

THERAPIST: Do you ever talk over body things with your body?

FRANKIE: That's a good idea. Like, I do get migraines and no part ever takes responsibility for that.

THERAPIST: Want to ask your body about it?

FRANKIE: Yes. (*Closes their eyes.*) Someone is saying, *Keep experimenting. The headaches are bad.*

THERAPIST: How do you understand that?

FRANKIE: Yeah. I got discouraged and gave up. My partner keeps encouraging me to try new things, but I don't. I guess I have a part who agrees with my partner.

THERAPIST: What kinds of things should you try?

FRANKIE: You know. Green light. Botox. Omega-3s. Stuff like that.

THERAPIST: So, no part of you claims responsibility for the headaches, but you're noticing a part who discouraged you from trying new things. Why did it discourage you?

FRANKIE: I guess it didn't want me to feel disappointed.

THERAPIST: How do you notice that part?

FRANKIE: Thoughts.

THERAPIST: How do you feel toward it?

● Cora Experiences Her Parts Kinesthetically and Aurally

THERAPIST: Do you see the anxious part?

CORA: No. I feel it in my stomach. And my shoulders get tense.

THERAPIST: How do you feel toward it?

CORA: I'd like to be a more relaxed person.

THERAPIST: What's the worst thing about being anxious?

CORA: I overthink everything and second-guess myself. Like, the minute I do something, I doubt my decision.

THERAPIST: So, thinking and doubting are features of your anxiety?

CORA: Well, maybe they're first and then comes the anxiety—in my stomach.

THERAPIST: Meaning there's a thinking/doubting part and an anxious part?

CORA: Yes.

THERAPIST: You hear the thinking/doubting part?

CORA: Yes.

THERAPIST: But you feel the anxious part.

CORA: Yes.

THERAPIST: Great. It's good for us to know how your parts communicate with you.

Frankie has a multisensory experience of her parts; Cora feels and hears her parts rather than seeing them. In my experience, the IFS approach to therapy is somewhat quicker and easier for clients if they are internally visual, but there's no right or wrong way to communicate inside. What's important is noticing and engaging with one's own experience. All of these examples illustrate some element of stage-setting as a way of facilitating therapy. They include winning permission to talk about parts in therapy, staying maximally experience-near with the client, and letting language guide you and the client toward releasing constraints rather than reinforcing old ones or putting more in place.

Conducting Sessions

1. Be aware of your language.

2. Is the client internally visual? If not, explore how they experience their parts and adjust your language accordingly. If they are visual, ask them to describe parts and notice their ages when a new part comes up.

3. If you're skeptical about the idea of little people living in the mind, suspend your disbelief and stay experience-near with your client's presentation. Schwartz (2017) calls parts *sacred inner beings*. They have their own brand of consciousness. They travel around in time, move in and out of the body, and can assume an endless variety of shapes. Each has its own feelings and developmental level. They live with us, they have experiences, they influence our behavior, and they make choices. Therefore, they can alter their behavior if they wish.

4. Talk with protectors before talking with exiles. If an exile comes up first, negotiate with it to wait until protectors give permission for contact.

5. Assert that exiled parts don't need to change, and reassure protectors that you're not trying to control or change them, either. Tell them you honor their work, and now you're offering the resources of the Self to them and the exiles they protect.

6. If firefighter parts are active, offer to help the manager part they're opposing.

7. If manager parts dominate from the get-go, offer to help them and the exile they protect.

8. Use the U-turn:
   - Continually guide the client to notice their parts.
   - Counter protective projections and interrupt protector monologues by guiding the client to notice the part who is speaking and ask about its motives. *What does this part want for you? What does it need from you?*
   - Praise protectors for their hard work and ask them to take a break to discuss their motives.
   - Use hypotheticals to propose options that protectors will reject out of hand as impossible.

9. Whenever you talk with a manager or a firefighter, ask about its fears, offer to address those fears, and ask if it's willing to meet the client's Self.

Prioritize Compassion

1. If a protector is not willing to meet the Self, talk with it directly while the client listens, elicit Self-energy from the client (if possible) with questions along the way (*How do you feel toward this part after hearing what it just said?*), and then ask again if the part is willing to meet the Self.
2. Stay focused on introducing protectors to the client's Self, guide the client's Self to address protector fears, identify exiled parts, and ask for permission to help them.
3. Ask clients to notice how they access Self on their own.

Watch for Polarities; Validate Both Sides

Every extreme protector is balanced by another protector. IFS calls this a polarity. When a proactive manager becomes extreme, a reactive firefighter steps in to create some balance. The manager disapproves of the firefighter's tactic and doubles down. The firefighter follows suit. These two parts become increasingly hostile toward one another and ever more extreme. If the client speaks from or about one protector, you can assume the opposing side is in the wings. Because we don't want shadow players in therapy, we get polarities out in the open by naming them. If we're just hearing about one side of a polarity, we guide the client to notice the other side. For example, we might guide the client to notice how they respond to excessive inhibition (*Do you ever rebel against all that responsibility?*). Or to notice how they respond to excessive disinhibition (*Do you ever feel concerned about watching TV all night?*). Then we validate the concerns of both sides, ask who they protect, and offer to help the exile.

● Ilsa's Polarity

Here is an example of how I might intervene with a polarity.

THERAPIST: So, I hear one team of parts browbeats you to stay at work late, be compulsively careful about your notes, go in on Saturday if you haven't finished everything, and so on. In general, this team makes you much slower and more thorough than your colleagues. In response, you have parts who are desperate for a break. They do things like keeping you up too late at night watching binge-worthy TV, urging you to eat a gummy of cannabis as soon as you get home so that you don't spend the evening fretting about work, and eating snacks for hours after dinner.

ILSA'S FEARFUL MANAGER: I feel trapped.

THERAPIST: I hear that.

ILSA'S FEARFUL MANAGER: I have to be thorough at work. I have no choice. My supervisor is pitiless.

THERAPIST: There's the proactive team.

ILSA'S REBELLIOUS FIREFIGHTER: I can't keep this up. I'm so tired I can't even get the basics done on weekends.

THERAPIST: Here's the other team. Let's get both teams together with you for a chat.

ILSA'S FEARFUL MANAGER: How?

THERAPIST: Invite them to meet you at an expandable conference table. You sit at the head so they can all see you. Now just notice who shows up. Let me know when everyone's there.

ILSA'S FEARFUL MANAGER: (*A long pause.*) Okay.

THERAPIST: Do they see you?

ILSA'S FEARFUL MANAGER: No. They're arguing.

THERAPIST: Ask them to stop for a moment and look at you. (*She nods.*) How do they respond?

ILSA'S FEARFUL MANAGER: They're quiet.

THERAPIST: Let them know we've been listening and we're aware that both sides have valid concerns. Will they let you help?

ILSA'S FEARFUL MANAGER: They want to know who I am.

THERAPIST: What do you say?

ILSA'S FEARFUL MANAGER: (*Shrugs.*) I don't know.

THERAPIST: Ask the part who's standing in for you to scoot over and sit next to you. Then ask for a volunteer who would like to find out more about you.

ILSA'S EXILE: Okay. The one in the suit.

THERAPIST: Ask the one in the suit to look you in the eye and let you know who they see there.

ILSA'S EXILE: She sees a scared little girl.

THERAPIST: Ask the scared little girl to scoot over and sit right next to you on the other side. Then ask the suit to look again. Who does she see now?

ILSA: Someone she doesn't know.

THERAPIST: How does the part respond to that person?

ILSA: She seems uncomfortable. She's afraid I won't need her.

THERAPIST: What do you say?

ILSA: We can work it out. I'm fair.

THERAPIST: Who does she protect?

ILSA: The little girl.

THERAPIST: Ask everyone at the table to look at you now. Would she, and all the other parts here, be willing to let you help the little girl?

The arc of this interchange covers the client describing a very common polarity (an overbearingly anxious managerial team vs. a reactive firefighter team that provides relief), her polarized protectors meeting her Self, and our conversation becoming an inquiry about her exile. Getting polarized protectors to pay attention to the client's Self and unblend enough to answer questions about the exile they protect can take a lot longer than this segment of a session illustrates. The byword is patience. For an example of how to encourage cooperation among teams of protectors who are estranged and hostile, see the treatment tips in Chapter 13.

Polarity Ping-Pong

When a client speaks in back-to-back contradictions, you are watching a ping-pong match between their protectors. Here is an example. Devon is 18 years old and came to therapy at his parents' insistence.

DEVON'S MANAGER: I want my parents to be involved in my therapy.

THERAPIST: Okay. Sign this release of information and I'll call them.

DEVON'S FIREFIGHTER: (*After reading the ROI.*) I wouldn't sign this if you paid me. I'm 18 years old. What I do is none of their business.

Although I want Devon's Self to get in on this conflict, the parts go back and forth, one blending and then the other, and the client's Self is not accessible. So being a sportscaster and calling their match, I keep inviting the client's Self to be present. The client's Self will ultimately be their referee.

THERAPIST: I hear one part who wants the parents involved and one part who doesn't.

DEVON'S MANAGER: I do think they should be involved.

THERAPIST: That's one part.

DEVON'S FIREFIGHTER: Over my dead body.

THERAPIST: There's the other part. Are you there, Devon? Do you hear these two parts? They have a big disagreement.

We can invite the client to notice protector ping-pong matches and help the client to start intervening on a regular basis by saying something like: *I hear you both. You each have an important point. Will you let me help?*

EXERCISE

Is This Protector Focused on Another Protector or an Exile?

One extreme will always be matched by another. To reveal either a polarized protector or an exile, ask the target protector, *What would happen if you stopped doing what you do?* It might say something like the following:

- *If he's not pleasing, he'll look selfish and alienate everyone.*
- *If she's not assertive, she'll look weak.*
- *If he has needs, he'll be rejected.*
- *If she's not nice, she'll be angry.*

Write down what you hear and ask if this protector is willing to let the client's Self help the part (it will be an exile or a polarized protector) who it is describing. If so, set an intention to take that inquiry up in your own therapy. If not, ask the part if it's willing to explain its concerns and write those down as a starting place for further inquiry.

EXERCISE

Intervening in Manager–Firefighter Polarities

Managerial shaming fuels shameless firefighter behaviors. Therefore, when there is a manager–firefighter polarity, it's a good idea to start by focusing on the manager.

1. Identify a firefighter behavior and notice the manager's concern. You can choose a firefighter behavior that is relatively low key—*I just eat a lot of healthy foods at night, you know? The problem is, I munch for hours while I watch TV*—or it can be high profile and costly—*I've been binge drinking and driving. I have to stop.*

2. Talk to the manager:
   What would happen if you stopped shaming the part who drinks?
   What if the Vincenzo-who's-not-a-part could help the drinking part?
   Whom do you protect?
   Would you be willing to meet the Vincenzo-who's-not-a-part?

What if the Vincenzo-who's-not-a-part could help the one you protect?

Thank the manager for having this chat and ask if it's okay for you to talk with the firefighter.

3. Now ask the firefighter some questions:

   What would happen if you stopped drinking?

   What if the Vincenzo-who's-not-a-part could help the [manager] part who criticizes (or, who, for another example, works too hard)?

   Whom do you protect?

   Would you be willing to meet the Vincenzo-who's-not-a-part?

   What if the Vincenzo-who's-not-a-part could help the one you protect?

Thank the firefighter and ask both of these parts to sit down with you. Ask if they listened to each other. Tell them you can help the parts they protect so they won't have to work so hard and be so extreme. Ask if they are interested. Ask for their permission to help the exile(s) they protect. Ask them to describe their exile(s) and set the intention to help that part or those parts. (For a description of helping exiles, see Chapter 11.)

Honor Wary Parts

The quickest route to a firefighter's heart is respect, which speaks to their pivotal role as shame protectors. Here is an example. Jamal, a 40-year-old cisgender, married, gay, African American man, was reluctant to engage in therapy with a White European American therapist.

● Jamal Isn't Sure

Jamal's parts were divided between managers who wanted to accede to his brother's recommendation that he come to see me and managers who thought this was a bad idea. Although he was not committed to following through, Jamal came to an initial session to talk about trying therapy at his brother's insistence because he was drinking heavily after retiring from the army.

JAMAL'S FIREFIGHTER: John thinks I'm drinking too much.

THERAPIST: Do you agree?

JAMAL'S FIREFIGHTER: I don't get the bottle out till the sun goes down, and I never drink alone. My husband drinks with me. Though, it's true, not as much as me.

THERAPIST: So, you disagree with your brother?

[*I try again to learn how the presenting part views Jamal's drinking.*]

JAMAL'S FIREFIGHTER: I was in the service for 20 years. I've been all over the world. John is an accountant who lives where we were born, in Philadelphia. We are different.

[*Again, the part doesn't answer.*]

THERAPIST: You and John have had different experiences, and you live differently now.

[*I give up on questioning the part and mirror it instead.*]

JAMAL'S MANAGER: Our father was an alcoholic, and our mother committed suicide, so of course, he's worried about me.

[*Another part speaks.*]

THERAPIST: Did you come here today to reassure John?

JAMAL'S FIREFIGHTER: (*Looking at the therapist with a bit more interest.*) Yes.

THERAPIST: Can you say more?

JAMAL'S FIREFIGHTER: I knew you were White, but John urged me to see you anyway. Now that I'm sitting here, I'm not sure it's a good idea. (*A short silence.*) Does that make you uncomfortable?

THERAPIST: No. I'm a White person in America and I'm aware that White people are often ignorant and hurtful to people who are not White. That said, if you want to try this out with me, I will be aware of my parts and listen to myself—and make a repair if I screw up.

JAMAL'S FIREFIGHTER: What if I challenge you?

THERAPIST: I hope you would if you felt the need. My job in that case would be to help my own parts relax and stand back so I can guide you in getting to know your internal system.

JAMAL'S FIREFIGHTER: My internal system?

THERAPIST: The idea of this approach to therapy is that we all have subpersonalities, or parts. A community inside the mind. For example, you have a part who isn't so sure that John's concern about your drinking is valid, and it also wasn't sure you should proceed with a White therapist. And then I heard another part—the one who understands John's reasons for being concerned about you, given your family history.

JAMAL'S MANAGER: (*Looks at therapist for a while.*) Say more.

THERAPIST: About?

JAMAL'S MANAGER: This kind of therapy.

THERAPIST: First can I ask you something? (*Jamal nods.*) Have you been in therapy before?

JAMAL'S FIREFIGHTER: Yes. My boss sent me to therapy after I hit my brother-in-law's boyfriend. He was a violent man. I told him I'd kill him if he ever touched my brother-in-law again. So he left. (*Smiles.*) Trey is still mad at me. I'm not sorry.

THERAPIST: What was your experience of therapy?

JAMAL'S FIREFIGHTER: I don't have an anger problem. I have an allergy to violent men.

THERAPIST: Violent men?

JAMAL'S FIREFIGHTER: I get the irony.

THERAPIST: No, it was a real question. Have you been hurt by violent men?

JAMAL'S FIREFIGHTER: My father never hit me or John. But he beat my mother when he was drinking.

THERAPIST: I see.

JAMAL'S FIREFIGHTER: *I* am violent.

THERAPIST: I hear that.

JAMAL'S FIREFIGHTER: But I'm not like my father. I don't become violent because I drink. I drink to avoid being violent.

THERAPIST: Alcohol puts a damper on an angry part of you? (*Jamal nods.*) If you choose to do this, I can show you how to help your angry part and the parts it protects. But before we go further, I want to be clear about what I do and don't mean by *help*. I don't mean I'll show you how to control or change your parts. I do mean we would explore what they fear, what they're mad about, and what they need.

JAMAL: Thank you for saying that.

THERAPIST: And if you want to try this approach but with a Black therapist, I'll help you look for someone.

JAMAL: I'll think about it. My brother suggested you.

THERAPIST: Okay. But if we proceed, that offer remains. If you ask, I'll help.

JAMAL: (*Jokingly.*) Do I have to talk about parts?

THERAPIST: You don't have to do anything. But if you don't mind, I'll talk about parts.

JAMAL: Okay, I'll give it a try. Here goes. One part of me is relieved at the idea of talking to someone. Other parts will never trust a White person.

THERAPIST: In this kind of therapy, we say all parts are welcome. So your wary and angry parts are welcome here.

JAMAL: Yeah. They don't believe you.

THERAPIST: Fair enough. Let me say one more thing. You're not here to educate me about race in America, or White aggression or microaggressions, but you will be educating me about you. Do I have your permission to ask questions if I'm not sure I understand your experience? (*He nods.*) I also have one request. When I disappoint one of your parts, will they please tell you so that you can let me know?

JAMAL: Who am *I* in all this?

THERAPIST: That's what I want to show you.

I think of IFS therapy as occurring in a theatre that has, as theatres typically do, two sets of doors. The first set opens into the lobby from the outside world, the second set opens into the theatre itself. Many clients who start therapy have only agreed to step into the lobby. Their parts are not ready to go inside and see what's happening on the lighted stage in their psyche. This is particularly true for people who feel mandated to therapy or want help but for some reason can't choose a preferred helper. But it can also be true of a client like Jamal who was urged to try a particular therapist but would not have chosen to go to therapy on his own and certainly would not have chosen a White European American. Nonetheless, Jamal had parts in the wings who shared his brother's concerns, so he took his brother's advice.

Some clients want a therapist who shares certain qualities. For example, they want help from someone who speaks the same mother tongue, who looks like them, or who has been subjected to a certain category of negative experience such as racism, homophobia, or transphobia. At the same time, some clients don't feel that way. It's important to ask. In either case, as I've been saying, therapy can't go forward without the fuel of willingness. It's crucial to listen to parts who have concerns and invite them to keep speaking up.

If a client tries therapy with you and clearly does not want you for a therapist, you can only offer to do your best to help them look elsewhere (you have access to listservs and other networks that they don't) for someone who meets their criteria. Sometimes an individual's options are severely limited, sometimes not. In an ideal world, people would be guaranteed choice and would have plenty of options, but the process of accessing psychotherapy can be far from ideal. People who pay out of pocket have the most choice, in theory, but can have trouble finding a therapist who meets their particular criteria or lives in their geographical area. People who use health insurance to see a therapist privately may have some choice of therapist. And people who seek help at a mental health center or a hospital are often assigned to a therapist and have no choice at all. If we do our job skillfully, we can probably help regardless of the client's circumstances.

Setting the Stage for Therapy

Listen for Shaming and Guilting

- The client shames themself.
- The client shames someone else.
- The client expresses adaptive guilt directly.
- The client expresses maladaptive guilt indirectly.

Talk about Parts

- Listen to stories, but talk parts.
- If a client objects to talking about parts, you can use their language.
- Or ask them to try your language.
- Or try making a deal: You say *feelings*, I'll say *parts*.

Notice Your Language

- Try avoiding the word *change*.

Clarify the Client's Language

- What does *I feel sad* mean?
- What does *I understand* mean?
  - To find out, just have the client tell the part what they understand and let the part decide if they've got it right.

Assess the Client's Sensory Experience

- Is it visual, kinesthetic, or aural?

Honor Wary Parts

- How willing are the client's protectors to go on this journey with you as the guide?
  - Did this client choose you?
  - Do their parts have concerns about your intentions and abilities?
    - Are they worried that you will be ignorant?
    - Are they worried that you will inevitably be biased?
    - Are they worried because people who look like you are routinely, intentionally or unintentionally, shaming?

Watch for Polarities; Validate Both Sides

- Polarities are always there. Listen for them. Don't take a side. This can be easier said than done.

Conclusion

I've made some suggestions that aim to lay the groundwork for therapy, including tracking your own Self-energy, listening for shaming and guilting as the client talks, being aware of your language, asking your client how they notice and experience their parts, noticing protector polarities from first contact and validating both sides, and checking with new clients on real-world concerns and constraints that may govern the willingness of their protectors to engage in therapy. It's not that therapy is impossible if a client has unwilling parts; it's that you'll need to woo unwilling parts to make therapy possible, probably by talking with them directly.

CHAPTER 9

Unblend

Different therapies have different ways of helping clients get emotional distance from daunting events. Eye movement desensitization and reprocessing (EMDR), for example, instructs clients to see traumatic experience as a movie. In IFS, we want a little distance and a lot of connection, which makes live theatre a good metaphor for what we do. I think of therapy as improvisational theatre with parts, and I often talk about parts being onstage, in the spotlight, or in the wings. The theatre has a lobby, seating for the audience, a stage, and everything backstage. If the client will only go as far as the lobby when therapy starts, we hang out there and talk about going into the theatre. When their parts are ready to begin the show, we go in. But in this theatre the lights only go up for the client. The stage is peopled with their parts. I sit in the dark, acting as the Self for our collective system entirely by feel and report until the client's Self takes over. All I can do is be curious about motives. Generally, the client tells me what parts are saying and doing, but not always. In any case, I have just one goal: I want them to acknowledge the client's Self. If they won't, I talk with them until they will. When they will, I talk with the client's Self, who talks with them.

Blending and Unblending

When vulnerable parts are included, protectors cooperate, the Self leads, and the theatre of the mind functions well. But if there is no Self to lead and protective parts (or teams of them) compete, the mind becomes chaotic. Blended protectors hold forth, hogging the spotlight. Other protectors mill about in the wings or backstage. And vulnerable parts, who were excluded long ago, are an ever-present subterranean force, whether hiding in a corner, wailing in a basement, or hammering on the back door. This mental disarray in the absence of internal leadership is the result of protectors having spent years denying, discounting, sidestepping, or bypassing the person's actual experience. We compound this mistake if we ignore their motives. As we guide clients to pay attention internally with respect and curiosity, they may feel shivers of anxiety (managers shun risk) or dread (inner inquiry can unleash critics, exiles, or disinhibited firefighters), yet, because all parts need attention, many will perk up.

The more the client can observe and describe their parts, the more their parts will take notice and cooperate. We can, as Schwartz teaches, achieve what Dan Siegel (2018) calls the *window of tolerance*—a regulated nervous system—by helping extreme parts unblend (Schwartz & Sweezy, 2020). Protectors who fight to control consciousness are not ready to cooperate, but if they feel safe they do actually want to be in relationship. When they first unblend, they are testing for safety. If a protector, for example, agrees to let the Self talk with another part, it's experimenting with being relational and testing to see if the Self can be trusted. Our job is to pass the test.

When Protectors Unblend, Everyone Can Feel

Feelings, like the starry night sky for early navigators, offer direction. When we have choices, feelings tell us what to choose. What do I want for breakfast? Who do I want to marry? Protective parts obscure that compass with their activities—avoidance, denial, distraction, dissociation, suppression, erasure, and so on. We feel lost when those activities cloud the mind; when they stop, we get direction again. There is plenty of room for all parts and feelings in the inner multiverse; it functions best as a lively, interactive, expansive space. Here is an example of a client who is just beginning to be able to notice and get direction from her feelings.

● Eliza Notices Herself

Eliza was a 19-year-old, cisgender, single, Korean American college student with a history of anxiety and depression.

ELIZA'S MANAGER: I want to be less anxious.
[*This blended part is talking to me about the anxious part. The client's Self is not yet in evidence.*]
THERAPIST: You're concerned about a part who feels anxious.

[I speak to the blended part directly without stopping to say that I'm speaking to a part.]

ELIZA'S MANAGER: The anxiety gets in the way of practically everything!

[The blended part complains again about the other part.]

THERAPIST: You are the part of Eliza who wants to do something about this anxiety.

[I switch to speaking about Eliza to the blended part in the third person.]

ELIZA'S MANAGER: Yes.

[By not disagreeing, the blended part endorses the idea that it is just one part of Eliza.]

THERAPIST: How long have you been worried about the anxiety?

[I continue speaking with the blended part.]

ELIZA'S MANAGER: Since she was a little girl.

[The blended part now starts speaking about Eliza in the third person and names an exile.]

THERAPIST: You've been trying to help Eliza with anxiety since she was little. How has it been going?

[I interview the blended part.]

ELIZA'S MANAGER: As you see, I'm here.

[The blended part admits feeling defeated.]

THERAPIST: There's another Eliza who is not the anxious part. She could help you. Would you like to meet her?

ELIZA'S MANAGER: Okay.

THERAPIST: Look Eliza in the eye. Who do you see?

ELIZA'S MANAGER: An anxious girl.

THERAPIST: Okay. I'll speak with the anxious girl and you can listen. (*She nods.*) Are you there? (*Eliza nods.*) Would you be willing to move over and sit next to Eliza so everyone can see you and her? (*Eliza nods.*) Thanks. Now I'll talk again with the one who doesn't like the anxiety. Are you there? (*Eliza nods.*) Look Eliza in the eye again. Who do you see now?

[First I ask the exile to sit next to Eliza so the manager part can see both of them, then I ask the manager to look again.]

ELIZA: It says, *Where have you been?*

[The manager part has now seen Eliza's Self, which caused it to unblend.]

THERAPIST: What do you say, Eliza?

ELIZA: What can I say?

THERAPIST: It is a puzzle, isn't it? You didn't mean to leave your parts alone, and they didn't deserve to be left alone. But now that you're here you can help the anxious part. Would that be good?

[*I address Eliza's Self directly.*]

ELIZA: Yes.

THERAPIST: How do you feel toward the anxious part now, Eliza?

[*This Geiger-counter question tells us how much access the client has to their Self.*]

ELIZA: (*A long pause in which she looks increasingly lost.*) What?

THERAPIST: What happened?

ELIZA: I spaced out.

[*A dissociative part—a reactive firefighter—took over, most likely because it was afraid of Eliza being in contact with the anxious exile.*]

THERAPIST: Ask the part who took you out just now why it jumped in.

[*Of necessity, this dissociative part becomes our new target for the moment.*]

ELIZA: No answer.

[*We have no relationship with the dissociative part yet, and it may, in any case, be preverbal.*]

THERAPIST: Do you see it?

ELIZA: It rolls in like fog.

THERAPIST: How do you feel toward it?

Note that the dissociative part was ready to jump in quickly if we made a move toward the anxious exile. Dissociative parts don't explain themselves; they take control. The therapist can talk with a dissociative part and ask it to be direct about its concerns, but it may require coaxing, repetition, patience, and time to form a relationship with a dissociative part.

What Are Suicide Parts Doing?

Suicide parts can be proactive and soothing (*Don't worry! There's always a way out*) or reactive and dangerous (*Now is the time to die*). Here is an example.

● Rui's Risk

Rui was a 29-year-old single, gender-nonbinary, Portuguese American who came to therapy complaining of social isolation and hypersensitivity in relationships.

Rui's Manager: I can't stand to disappoint anyone. I'm embarrassed to say that I start to think about killing myself if someone looks disappointed.

Therapist: How do you feel toward the part who can't stand to disappoint?

Rui's Manager: Very close.

[*That is, the part is blended.*]

Therapist: You mean spatially or emotionally?

Rui's Manager: Spatially. (*Pats the left side of their head.*) It's here.

Therapist: What happens to it when someone seems disappointed?

Rui's Manager: I panic and I can't think about anything else. I wake up in the night and can't stop thinking about whatever happened. And then this other part says, *Well, this would be a good time to die.*

Therapist: What's happening when you can't think about anything else?

Rui's Manager: A voice yells at me.

Therapist: Whose voice?

Rui's Manager: My father's.

Therapist: What does his voice yell?

Rui's Manager: That I'm making mistakes. I'm bad.

Therapist: Is that one of your parts using his voice, or is it him acting inside you?

Rui: It's my part.

Therapist: Is it yelling at you now? (*Rui nods.*) Would it be willing to stop and tell us what the worry is?

Rui's Hammer: The worry is that I'm an idiot—

Therapist: (*Interrupting.*) I know this part is good at its job. But we want to know why it does the job. Would it take a few minutes now and do something different? (*After a pause, Rui nods.*) Can you see it, Rui?

Rui: It's a hammer.

Therapist: Is the hammer willing to say what's important about being a hammer?

Rui's Hammer: I have to be perfect.

Therapist: What happens if you aren't perfect?

Rui's Hammer: I usually am.

Therapist: But what happens if you're not?

Rui's Hammer: Everyone suffers.

Therapist: And then what?

RUI'S HAMMER: It's bad.

THERAPIST: Who is *everyone*?

RUI: My father is mad and my mother gets upset, and then my sisters act up, and then their teachers are unhappy . . .

THERAPIST: A domino effect. (*Rui nods.*) Can we be curious about this? (*Rui nods.*) When you're not perfect, everyone suffers. What happens inside you?

RUI: Despair.

THERAPIST: And what do you believe about yourself?

RUI: I'm not up to it.

THERAPIST: And then what happens?

RUI: It feels like it would be easier to die.

THERAPIST: How does the hammer feel about that?

RUI: It wants me to be perfect, not dead. It hammers harder.

THERAPIST: So, has it succeeded in making you perfect?

RUI: Ha ha.

THERAPIST: Is it tired? (*Rui nods.*) Would it be interested in an experiment? It could put the hammer down for a bit and meet with you and the suicide part.

[*Include reactive firefighter parts, especially suicide parts.*]

RUI: (*Considers.*) Okay.

THERAPIST: Meet them at a conference table.

RUI: Okay.

THERAPIST: Do they see you? (*Rui nods.*) Are they ready to talk? (*Rui nods.*) How do you feel toward the hammer now?

[*I continue to focus on the critic who drives this dynamic. The suicide part is reacting to the hammer's criticisms.*]

RUI: It's not helping.

THERAPIST: And given that it's not helping, how do you feel toward it? (*Rui shrugs.*) Is it okay to be curious? (*Rui nods.*)

THERAPIST: Who does it protect?

[*I ask about the hammer's motive.*]

RUI: Me, it says.

[*This means the hammer doesn't see Rui as an adult. It may view itself as protecting the whole system, or it may protect one exile.*]

THERAPIST: How old does it think you are?

RUI: All ages.

[*This is the exile.*]

THERAPIST: When did it get the job?

RUI: I was 6 or 7 maybe.

THERAPIST: Does that make sense to you? (*Rui nods.*) Ask this kid to sit next to you so the hammer and the suicide part can see who you really are.

Rui's suicide part came on the heels of despair, the feeling of an exile who was reacting to an inner critic, the hammer. I always ask critics if they're succeeding. Sometimes they cite small victories, but mostly they admit feeling unsuccessful and tired, which is our opportunity to offer help. In contrast, firefighter parts, like Rui's suicide part, are just concerned with short-term results. They will only consider the long-term costs of their behavior if they believe the client's Self can handle the feelings that recruit them to their jobs in the first place. For this reason, we want firefighters to watch as the client's Self asks managers to dial down, and we want both managers and firefighters to see that the client's Self can help the exile. If the manager says it will only dial down if the firefighter does, we negotiate a simultaneous de-escalation (Krause, Rosenberg, & Sweezy, 2017).

Unblending and Willingness

All parts can unblend, but they have to be willing. It's important to remember that they always have reasons, and we have a job, which is to discover and address their reasons effectively and respectfully. That said, protectors often cite habit as a way of maintaining the status quo. Habit, as I discuss elsewhere, is not a protector concern; it's a protective cover for concerns that have not yet been addressed adequately. Here is an example.

Adam Isn't Ready

Adam, a 59-year-old Moldovan Jewish American, had a protector who put him to sleep whenever an inquiry got close to the time of his mother's death from a stroke, which he witnessed when he was 4 years old.

THERAPIST: Would the sleepy part be willing to separate and let you help the 4-year-old, Adam?

ADAM'S SLEEPY PART: (*Eyes drooping.*) It can't.

THERAPIST: Would it let you be awake if we agreed not to approach the 4-year-old right now?

ADAM'S SLEEPY PART: (*Closing his eyes.*) Hmmm. Maybe that's a good idea.

THERAPIST: It's a deal. Take your time.

ADAM: (*Leans over, head in hands, and rubs his scalp, then shakes his head and sits up, eyes open.*) Okay.

THERAPIST: Are you here?

ADAM: I'm coming back.

THERAPIST: I want the sleepy part to know that it can be direct with us. It can say no. We won't go to the 4-year-old without its permission. Okay? (*Adam nods.*) But here's one thing you should know. The sleepy part can let you stay present and awake if it decides that would be safe.

ADAM: How do you know?

THERAPIST: Are you always sleepy? (*Adam shakes his head.*) Do you fall asleep uncontrollably?

ADAM: No.

THERAPIST: You don't normally fall asleep during the day out of the blue? (*Adam shakes his head.*) So, the sleepy part is choosing to put you to sleep sometimes. I trust it has a good reason. But if you could help the 4-year-old safely without being emotionally overwhelmed, would it still need to put you to sleep?

ADAM: (*Pause.*) I fell asleep all the time when I was a kid, so they put me in therapy.

THERAPIST: The sleepy part has done this for a long time.

ADAM: It's not sure it can change.

THERAPIST: How old is it?

ADAM: Five.

THERAPIST: If it didn't have to put you to sleep any more, what would it rather do?

ADAM: Play.

THERAPIST: The sleepy part puts you to sleep to keep the 4-year-old out of mind, but if the 4-year-old felt better, the sleepy part could play instead. Would it like to meet you first and decide if that's a good plan? We could do that without going anywhere near the 4-year-old.

ADAM: (*Attends inside for a few beats.*) Yes.

Extreme protectors can (and do) share the spotlight with other parts all the time. Adam, for example, did not fall asleep in just any situation. People in the grip of a disinhibition (falling asleep, using substances, dissociating, bingeing and purging, having temper tantrums) can often still function in school, hold a job, make dinner, exercise, bring up kids, paint paintings, make music, write books, and so on. So, if a part says it can't unblend, don't take that literally, but do appreciate that it has a reason for not wanting to unblend. If its reason seems invalid in the current context of the client's life (Adam's Self could actually take care of his 4-year-old), remember that it was valid in the past and that this protector may still be living in the past with the exile.

Unblending and the Firefighter Hierarchy

Firefighters are reactive and often impulsive or compulsive, but they're not all dangerous. The urge to go for a walk in the middle of a work day, the reminder when you're digging in the garden and getting too hot that you will soon get on your bike and sail in the breeze, the pleasure of eating a meal after the labor of cooking it—our firefighter parts balance *wants* to *shoulds*. The more a society (or an individual on their own) leans into *shoulds*, the harder firefighters work to represent their other needs. And when managers get panicky and critical about this, firefighters respond commensurately, upping the ante. If binge-watching TV isn't a sufficient distraction from managerial shaming, the next rung up might be binge eating while watching TV, drinking, cruising a bar to pick up a sexual partner, and so on. At the top of this ladder, we find suicide. Here is an example.

● Ian's Despair

Ian is a 50-year-old single, cisgender, Scottish American man with a gambling habit. He had moved from the East Coast to the outskirts of Los Angeles as a young man and had spent much of his life trekking in the wilderness, at first picking up odd jobs to support his passion, eventually becoming a paid guide.

IAN: (*Head in hands.*) I drove to Nevada and spent the weekend betting again.

THERAPIST: Why now?

IAN: It's 115 degrees in Oregon. Animals are dying in droves. California is on fire. The Los Angeles sky is apocalypse orange. Why shouldn't I have fun?

THERAPIST: Was it fun?

IAN: Well, I kept looking for a tree to drive into on the way home. But I didn't want to hurt any trees. Heck, I didn't even want to hurt a concrete overpass!

THERAPIST: Ian, you have some parts with strong ideas about how to help you when things look this bad in the world.

IAN: Yes.

THERAPIST: How do you feel toward the gambling and suicide parts now?

IAN: Sometimes it's unbearable to be human.

THERAPIST: What's the most unbearable thing for you?

IAN: We are doing this. We are choosing this. Doesn't that blow your mind? How could we possibly be sleepwalking into collective suicide?

THERAPIST: The gambling part distracts from your astonishment and sadness? (*Ian nods.*) Can we get permission to help the sad part?

IAN: Yes.

THERAPIST: Where do you notice it?

IAN: In my heart.

Ian is not in denial about catastrophic climate events. As he takes stock of the disaster for the land and the wildlife he loves, he feels astonished and sad. My job is to help him connect with and comfort his sad part so that his firefighters don't take over and bankrupt or kill him. To live with and respond to this extreme challenge, he needs fortitude and comfort.

Unblending and the Persuasion of Exiles

When an exile blends, other parts feel overwhelmed. Strong feelings are the reason protectors banished the exile in the first place. They couldn't challenge its beliefs because they agreed, and they couldn't help the exile calm down because its feelings were contagious. As a result, they've aimed to suppress or distract from the exile's strong feelings. In contrast, the client's Self does not endorse any crippling identity beliefs (*I'm worthless*, and so on) and is not afraid of strong feelings. The Self is a calming counter force, a ballasted boat in rough waters. We can help exiles unblend even when they've taken over completely. As Schwartz (2017) says, we don't do this by teaching the client cognitive or distracting skills that will put the exile out of mind; we do it by inviting the exile to separate, stick around, and meet the Self. Here is an example.

● Selma's Fears

Selma was a 25-year-old cisgender, single, German American woman who grew up in dangerous circumstances. Sometimes a terrified exile would blend during therapy.

THERAPIST: Can you hear me, Selma? (*She is cringing, hands over her head.*) I see that something terrible is happening to some part of you right now. I'm going to talk to the part directly. Okay? Selma and I are right here with you, and if you make a little space inside, Selma will help. Will you make room for her?

SELMA'S SCARED PART: (*A small voice.*) I don't know her.

THERAPIST: Would you like to know her? She can help. (*Selma nods.*) You're welcome here with us. I know other parts try to drive you away, but the Selma-who's-not-a-part can take care of you. Can you see her?

SELMA'S SCARED PART: Help!

THERAPIST: We're going to help you. I'm going to check with Selma for a minute. Are you there, Selma?

SELMA: A little.

THERAPIST: You're listening? (*Selma nods.*) Good. I'm going to talk with this scared part again. Are you there? (*Selma nods.*) Selma tells me you're making a little room for her. She's the one who can take care of you. Do you notice her now? (*Selma nods.*) You two can be together right now so you can feel her and she can feel you. (*Selma's hands come down slowly and she buries her face.*) Are you with the scared part now, Selma? (*Selma shakes her head no.*) Okay, I'll talk with it again. Are you there? (*Selma nods slightly.*) You deserve help. It's awful to feel alone when you're scared. We're just going to be here with you. How close do you want Selma to be?

SELMA'S SCARED PART: (*A small voice.*) Over there.

THERAPIST: Okay. Selma can you be over there?

SELMA: Yes.

THERAPIST: Can you see the scared part?

SELMA: Yes.

THERAPIST: Can she see you?

SELMA: If she looked up.

THERAPIST: Well, she doesn't have to do anything. We'll just be here with her.

SELMA: (*After a long pause.*) She relaxed a little.

THERAPIST: Stay with her.

SELMA: (*After another long pause.*) She looked up.

THERAPIST: How does she respond?

SELMA: She says where have I been.

THERAPIST: What do you say?

SELMA: I don't know.

THERAPIST: It is a mystery. When protective parts take over it can be like you don't exist. Yet when those parts are ready, there you are. You've been there all the time because you're always there. You can take care of this little one.

SELMA: What makes protective parts ready?

THERAPIST: Well, you notice them, so they notice you, and they understand that you intend to help scared, sad parts. If this little one is willing to be patient for a bit longer, you can talk with the protectors about letting you help her. Would she like to go to a safe place to wait for you?

SELMA: What if she isn't patient?

THERAPIST: She doesn't have to *feel* patient, she just has to *be* patient. If that's hard, she can ask for help.

SELMA: But what if she makes a mistake?

THERAPIST: Mistakes tell us what we need to practice. Let's practice with her right now. Here's a shorthand way of being separate but together. Put a volume dial, like from a stereo, on the table. It goes from 1 to 10 and controls how much she shares her feelings with you. It doesn't control her feelings, right? Just how much she shares her feelings with you right now. Okay? (*Selma nods.*) Tell her where to set the dial so you can stay with her.

SELMA: Two.

THERAPIST: Okay. Practice that and see how it feels.

SELMA: Better.

THERAPIST: If for some reason she turns the dial up and you disappear, she can turn it down again, because this dial goes up and down. As soon as she turns it down again, you'll be back, and she can explain why she turned it up. Is that a good arrangement? (*Selma nods.*) So much better than being alone. She has the power to make this happen. When protectors trust her not to overwhelm, they'll cooperate with you, and you'll be able to get back to her even faster. Is she willing to try that? (*Selma nods.*)

Out of all the parts who show up in therapy, exiles want help and are the most willing. But if an exile pushes for attention before protectors are ready, they just get more managerial shaming, firefighter disinhibition, and inner conflict. So, although we welcome them if they show up too soon, we also explain the problem and ask them to cooperate: *We're going to help you, but we can't do it without permission from those protectors. You can make this go faster by being patient. Are you willing to wait a little longer?*

Walking Polarized Parts Back from the Edge with Unblending

Therapies that aim to help chronically dysregulated clients now generally include a phase for practicing affect regulation skills similar to those Linehan developed for dialectical behavior therapy. In parts language, skills training offers the client tools to try something different. My view, as I expect is obvious by now, is that the client's ability to make use of these tools will depend on the willingness and cooperation of their protective parts. Less obvious, perhaps, is the matter of who will be responsible going forward. Do we still have protective parts after exiles unblend? If we don't need young parts to learn new skills, who will learn? In my experience, older, more capable managers who are waiting in the wings—and we all have plenty of them—activate when younger parts calm down. With the Self's co-regulating presence (or, as Linehan says, Wise Mind), an appropriate age hierarchy reasserts itself in the internal system, and older parts begin to bring all they have learned to the project of continuing to learn. They are the ones with the bandwidth and maturity to make use of new skills. Here are a few examples of how to help young protectors who are stuck in an unpleasant role or a high-conflict polarity to unblend, which makes way for older, more capable parts, as well as the client's Self.

● Anastasia's Disagreement

Anastasia, a 35-year-old, cisgender, heterosexual, European Roma American, had an extreme polarization and was experiencing whiplash between two serially blended protectors.

ANASTASIA'S MANAGER: I have to stop texting my boyfriend.

THERAPIST: You have a part who doesn't want you to text your boyfriend.

[*I start by translating her statement into parts language.*]

ANASTASIA'S FIREFIGHTER: Fuck him! He can't ghost me. He's got my stuff in his apartment.

[*A polarized part speaks.*]

THERAPIST: You also have a part who wants to text your boyfriend to get your stuff back.

[*I name the polarity.*]

ANASTASIA'S FIREFIGHTER: He's my ex-fucking boyfriend. Fuck him.

THERAPIST: You're the part who wants to text him.

[*As these parts are blending serially, I start calling the game.*]

ANASTASIA'S FIREFIGHTER: He cannot have my vinyl collection.

THERAPIST: You don't want him to keep your records.

ANASTASIA'S MANAGER: Well, I gave them to him.

THERAPIST: The other part points out that you gave them to him.

ANASTASIA'S FIREFIGHTER: That was a fucking mistake! A moment of weakness. A gesture. I was living there, too!

THERAPIST: You don't want him to have the records, and you are mad at him.

ANASTASIA'S MANAGER: He's not perfect, but he's a good person.

THERAPIST: You feel differently. The other part is mad, but you would give him the records. Do you hear these two parts, Anastasia? They disagree.

[*I name the polarity again and check for some awareness from Anastasia.*]

ANASTASIA'S FIREFIGHTER AND ANASTASIA'S MANAGER: He's not a good person. Good is what we *do*, not who we are. (*A pause.*) But good people sometimes do bad things.

[*The firefighter blends again. The manager counters.*]

THERAPIST: Do you hear them arguing, Anastasia?

[*I push for them to be co-conscious with Anastasia's Self.*]

ANASTASIA: (*A pause.*) Yes.

[*There she is.*]

THERAPIST: Do they notice you?

[*Now I can talk with her about her parts.*]

ANASTASIA: No.

THERAPIST: Ask if they're willing to notice you. (*Anastasia nods after a pause.*) Okay. Invite them to sit at a conference table with you. (*Anastasia nods.*) Do they see you?

ANASTASIA: They're glaring at each other. One of them has a dark suit on, like for work, and the other looks wild, hair in the air and cell phone in hand, ready to text.

THERAPIST: If you spoke to them, would they hear you?

ANASTASIA: Hard to tell.

THERAPIST: Let's try. Ask if they'd like some help.

ANASTASIA: Not a blink.

THERAPIST: Okay. Say you can help them get out of this precarious situation without abandoning either one of them.

ANASTASIA: That got a laugh.

THERAPIST: Are they willing to hear more? (*Anastasia nods.*) You can, in fact, help them both. If the one in the suit was willing to stop criticizing the one with the phone for just the last few minutes of our session, would the one with the phone be willing to put the phone on the table? (*A few beats, then she nods again.*) Great. Are they both willing to look at you now?

ANASTASIA'S FIREFIGHTER AND ANASTASIA'S MANAGER: Why should they?

THERAPIST: They can do it at the same time.

[*I address what I assume is an underlying fear of unilateral action rather than talking about how they would both benefit from unblending—but I could have done that instead.*]

ANASTASIA: Okay.

THERAPIST: Ask them to look you in the eye and tell you who they see.

ANASTASIA: A child.

THERAPIST: How old?

ANASTASIA: Nine.

[*This is the exile.*]

THERAPIST: Ask the 9-year-old to sit next to you and invite them to look again. Who do they see now?

ANASTASIA: They don't know me.

THERAPIST: You can help them both. Are they willing to check you out?

ANASTASIA: What do you propose?

In this example, I guide Anastasia to negotiate with polarized protectors who are in the middle of a high-tension, high-stakes disagreement. Crucially, I insist that Anastasia can help both sides. This gets a temporary truce and wins their attention long enough to introduce them to Anastasia's Self.

EXERCISE

An Unblending Game

This game aims to help parts get to know the Self and vice versa. Any part who wants to participate can; anyone who wants to watch can.

The Setup

- Picture a big space that will accommodate everyone who wants to play.
- This space is divided in two, like a basketball court.
- On one side, the client's Self faces toward the client's parts, who are on the other side.

The Self

- Next to the Self, who is dressed in a cloak of sunlight, is a big bin full of crystal balls that are filled with sunlight.

Parts

- The parts have their own bin full of crystal balls.
- They also have a tailor with many cloaks to hand out. Their cloaks come in all the colors of the rainbow.

The Game

We start the game with each part choosing a cloak and putting it on. Then they all take a crystal ball and put their chosen rainbow color in the ball, along with a private message for the Self. Meanwhile, the Self is putting a private message for each part in a sunlit crystal ball. We'll pause while they do that.

- Next, the Self and parts will exchange crystal balls.
- Parts will roll their crystal balls to the Self, who will take them in one by one, reflect on them, and send a sunlit crystal ball with a special message back to the part.
- Parts may want to hold the crystal balls from the Self, put them in their heart, or store them someplace. The balls are theirs to keep and absorb forever.
- When everyone has taken in their message, parts can circle up with the Self and hold hands.
- Parts who don't want to hold hands can be in the middle or outside or above the circle.
- Thank them.

Some Techniques That Facilitate Unblending

Helping parts to unblend is the key to making progress. Here are a number of effective techniques.

The Room

The first technique, *the Room*, is a great option when an exile threatens emotional overwhelm or a scary protector intimidates other parts. I used it with Eliot, a 29-year-old cisgender, single, gay Somali American man. Eliot's family fled the civil war in Somalia and came to the United States when he was 5 years old. He came to therapy because of nightmares and discovered a Kaiju.

ELIOT'S MANAGER: Do you know the Kaiju? (*I shake my head.*) It means *strange beast* in Japanese. It's like their version of Godzilla. This part is a Kaiju. Everyone inside is scared of him.

THERAPIST: Okay. Let's put him in a room that's safe and comfortable for him, and you be outside for now. Any part who doesn't want to watch you talking with the Kaiju can go to a waiting room.

ELIOT'S MANAGER: He hates being in the room. He's running around smashing into the walls.

THERAPIST: Ask him to take a break and tell you about himself.

ELIOT'S MANAGER: He says what do I want to know?

THERAPIST: What would you like to know about the Kaiju, Eliot?

ELIOT: Why are you trying to scare me?

THERAPIST: What does he say?

ELIOT: He wants a snack.

THERAPIST: What do Kaijus eat?

ELIOT: People.

THERAPIST: Ask if he belongs to you. Is he one of your parts?

ELIOT: Half and half.

THERAPIST: Some of his energy comes from outside you? (*Eliot nods.*) Are any of your other parts attached to the energy from outside? (*Eliot shakes his head no.*) Is he attached to it? (*Eliot nods.*) What would happen if he let it go?

ELIOT'S KAIJU: He won't.

THERAPIST: But if he did?

ELIOT'S KAIJU: I'd be weak and vulnerable.

THERAPIST: What if you could help your vulnerable parts so he didn't have to worry about them?

ELIOT: That would be great. But how am I going to do that?

THERAPIST: If the Kaiju is willing, I'll show you.

In this example, Eliot finds and begins to befriend a buffed-up firefighter part in the form of a Kaiju (Eliot was a big fan of Japanese manga). To speed this effort along, we put the Kaiju in a room so he could talk to it, and we sequestered the parts who were scared of it in a waiting room.

The Dial

When we're self-aware and compassionate, we know that we're inside of—inhabiting—the perspective of the Self. However, our parts have to be willing to unblend and let us get access to that perspective. If our parts unblend about 60%, we have a reasonable opening to communicate with them directly inside, though most people prefer 70% or more. The dial exercise, which I borrowed from hypnosis, is another way to help exiled parts who elicit protector backlash when they push for attention. As the following example illustrates, exiles will negotiate and can, given some attention and assistance, separate from the client's Self and from other parts. In the dial exercise, we ask the client and the exile to imagine a volume dial, like the one on a stereo system. This dial controls how intensely the exile shares its feelings with the client. If, for example, the dial is set at 2, the exile is 20% blended and 80% unblended. If client asks the exile to set the dial at 1 or 2 but the exile wants to set it higher, negotiate.

The dial works because protectors fear emotional overwhelming by exiles, and exiles are willing to negotiate not to overwhelm them as long as they know they're going to get attention. If the client's protectors are particularly fearful, set the dial low at first and practice going up and down. In this way protectors will see that the exile is more cooperative if it gets attention than if it's ignored. Here is an example.

● Jasmine's Exile Dials Down

Jasmine, a 32-year-old cisgender, married, Jamaican American lesbian, came to therapy looking for help with a long history of anxiety and depression. She had been in therapy for several months when this conversation took place.

JASMINE'S MANAGER: I'm afraid of getting overwhelmed. I have to, you know, function. I can't see you at 8:00 A.M. and go to work. But I also can't see you at 5:00 P.M. and sleep at night! Sometimes I think, "What have I done? Maybe I should have left all this alone."

THERAPIST: A part is telling you that you wouldn't be threatened with emotional overwhelm if you hadn't chosen to come to therapy right now?

JASMINE'S MANAGER: I know, I know. I was feeling bad.

THERAPIST: But this part is warning you that we're letting the cat out of the bag, right? (*Jasmine nods.*) Well, we actually want the cat out of that bag—safely. So let's talk about safety measures.

JASMINE'S MANAGER: Okay.

THERAPIST: If you could help the anxious part, would you be this depressed?

JASMINE: No.

THERAPIST: Does anyone object to you helping the anxious part?

JASMINE: (*Listens inside.*) No.

THERAPIST: Where do you notice it?

JASMINE: In my stomach.

THERAPIST: How do you feel toward it?

JASMINE'S MANAGER: I don't like it.

THERAPIST: Will the parts who don't like it let us talk with it about not overwhelming you?

JASMINE: Yes.

THERAPIST: How do you feel toward it now?

JASMINE'S MANAGER: I feel it too much.

THERAPIST: Okay. Ask if it's willing to begin getting some help right now? (*Jasmine nods.*) Okay, Jasmine, put it in a safe room and, for now, you stay outside the room. Give it a dial, like the volume dial on a stereo, that goes from one, which is low, to ten, which is high. This dial controls how much the anxious part shares its feelings with you. Where do you want it to set the dial so you can be present and not get overwhelmed?

JASMINE'S MANAGER: Two.

THERAPIST: Ask it to put the dial at two and see how that feels.

JASMINE: It thinks I'm telling it to go away.

THERAPIST: That's a reasonable misunderstanding. But we want just the opposite. If it shares the feelings with you at a level of two, other parts will relax, and you'll be more available.

JASMINE: Okay. It will try. (*After a minute of silence.*) Yes.

THERAPIST: How is that?

JASMINE'S MANAGER: Good. But what if it can't do this all the time?

THERAPIST: It was born with this skill. It can turn the dial down whenever it wants. Will there be any obstacle to turning the dial down?

JASMINE: When I feel alone, I get scared.

THERAPIST: The anxious part gets scared when it feels alone? (*Jasmine nods.*) You can help with that. Would it like help?

JASMINE'S ANXIOUS PART: Yes.

In this example, Jasmine starts off feeling anxious, which could come from an anticipatory manager part or an exile. Using the dial, she discovers that her exile is scared of being alone, and she offers to help.

Swap Perspectives

In another exercise, the Self sees through the eyes of a blended part and mirrors back what it sees. Then the Self invites the part to see through its eyes. This technique of swapping perspectives is simple but can be powerful. Here is an example.

● Arlo's Avatar Owns Up

Arlo, a 45-year-old cisgender, heterosexual, English Canadian man, was molested by a Catholic priest as a child. Although he speaks of having compassion for his parts, he is stalled in therapy. In this session, I conclude that a Self-like manager (I call them *avatar* parts) is blended, and I address it directly.

THERAPIST: I have the impression that a part may be standing in for you much of the time here in therapy.

ARLO'S AVATAR: Why do you think that?

THERAPIST: Because of how other parts respond. When you say you have compassion, they act as if you're trying to boss them around.

ARLO'S AVATAR: You mean I'm not me?

[*The Self-like part is blended and speaks directly here.*]

THERAPIST: You're a really important part of Arlo, but there's also an Arlo-who's-not-a-part that could help out. I know you work hard for Arlo, and it must be challenging when other parts, like the one who looks at porn, aren't cooperative.

[*I speak directly to the Self-like manager.*]

ARLO'S AVATAR: I have compassion for that boy, but porn is a disgusting habit! It has to stop.

[*He is referring to the exile (that boy), who actually turns his back when this Self-like manager tries to make contact.*]

THERAPIST: I know you feel that way, and I also know the porn part has its reasons. What if Arlo could mediate your disagreement with the porn part?

ARLO'S AVATAR: Who are you talking about?

THERAPIST: How old do you think Arlo is?

ARLO: He thinks I'm 9 years old.

[*Arlo speaks about this Self-like manager for the first time, indicating that it has unblended at least a bit.*]

THERAPIST: What do you say to him?

ARLO: I'm a grown-up. (*A pause.*) He's looking at me.

THERAPIST: How do you feel toward him?

[*As usual, I ask the Geiger-counter question to facilitate the relationship between Arlo's Self and his Self-like manager.*]

ARLO: I'd like to get to know him.

THERAPIST: How does he respond?

ARLO'S AVATAR: I am Arlo! I take care of him. What would he be without me?

[*The part claims to be Arlo but also describes what he does for Arlo.*]

THERAPIST: Are you there, Arlo?

ARLO: Yes.

THERAPIST: What do you say to him?

ARLO: I'm asking him and the boy to look in the mirror with me. (*A pause.*) He sees all three of us.

[*This is one way of sharing a new perspective.*]

THERAPIST: How old is he?

ARLO: He's nineteen. He knows he got me out of there. I know it, too. I'm grateful.

THERAPIST: Now it could be his turn. Would he like your help?

[*I turn the tables, suggesting that Arlo's Self can now help the manager.*]

ARLO: He wants to know what will happen to him. He doesn't want to disappear.

THERAPIST: He won't. He'll always be an important part of you. What would he like to do once you help the boy?

ARLO: He likes what he does.

THERAPIST: What do you say to him?

ARLO: Help me out, then.

THERAPIST: What does he need to hear from you?

ARLO: I wouldn't be alive without him. (*A few beats.*) He likes hearing that.

THERAPIST: Would he like to look at the boy through your eyes? (*Arlo nods.*) What's that like for him?

[*This is a way to offer protectors a new perspective on an exile.*]

ARLO: He's surprised.

THERAPIST: How does the boy respond?

ARLO: He turned around. (*A pause.*) He's saying thank you and I don't need your help anymore. He wants to stay with me.

THERAPIST: Okay with you?

ARLO: Yes.

THERAPIST: How does the 19-year-old respond?

ARLO: He's sad. He didn't mean any harm.

THERAPIST: Does the boy understand?

ARLO: Yes. He just doesn't want to be told what to do anymore.

THERAPIST: So, what needs to happen?

ARLO: You know, I have room for everyone.

THERAPIST: Would the boy like your help now? (*Arlo nods.*) How do you feel toward him?

This interaction illustrates how we can help parts swap or share perspectives. And there are lots of other options as well. We can, for example, invite the client to externalize parts into objects (little figures, stuffed animals, pillows, scarves, paper plates with drawings on them, etc.) and see from the object's (the part's) perspective, and then switch to see the part through the eyes of the Self. Or we can use the Gestalt technique of inviting the client to move around to different chairs or seats in a room. We can also invite the client to inhabit a part physically, with movement, posture, expression, and tone. In online sessions, we can invite them to represent different parts with different items of clothing.

Play

Young parts love to play, and all of the options mentioned earlier can be playful. Play is an inherently curious, engaged activity. I've said this before, but it bears repeating. Ask your skeptical parts to let you play with the following assumptions about who parts are.

1. Parts are like people; they have feelings, different developmental levels, and different roles to play within their own community.
2. Parts are also not like people because they can travel through time, adopt an endless variety of appearances, move around in the body, or leave it altogether.
3. Parts come online developmentally and then stay with us.
4. All protective parts aim to help.
5. Protective behavior is motivated and purposeful.
6. In contrast, exiles are largely reactive and motivated to get help.

● Josh Dares to Get His Way

The following example illustrates how each of these assumptions affect a therapist's interaction with a client's parts. Josh is 67-year-old, cisgender, heterosexual, Russian Jewish American widower. Two years after his wife died, he came to therapy saying he was depressed.

JOSH'S MANAGER: Sarah and I got together when we were sixteen. I was shy. She made friends, organized our social life, cooked, moved the furniture around, kept the kids going. She ran the PTO when they were in school. That's who she was. If I'd gone first, she'd be dating four different guys right now with a checklist to decide which was a keeper.

THERAPIST: What are your days like without her?

JOSH'S MANAGER: I retired when she got sick, so I'm not busy now. I lie in bed and wonder if I should get up. When I get up, I wonder if I should go downstairs.

THERAPIST: What's it like to lie in bed?

[*Note that this question is neutral. Although he did use the word* depression, *I don't assume he is describing something negative. At this point, I'm just curious about his internal experience.*]

JOSH: I like it. But then I think, *Shouldn't I have some purpose in life?* Maybe I should volunteer. Or maybe I should date.

THERAPIST: One part of you likes to lie in bed and another part wants you to volunteer or date.

JOSH: Yes.

THERAPIST: What's the best thing about lying in bed?

JOSH'S PLAYFUL PART AND HIS GUILTY PART: I'm free. I feel guilty saying that. Now that I think about it, I took advantage of Sarah. I let her handle things because she did it so well. Sometimes I even resented her. I feel bad about that.

THERAPIST: I hear different parts. You have parts who relied on Sarah's strengths, and a part who maybe felt overshadowed by her at times. That part may be enjoying this opportunity to lie around in bed. Do you think? (*Josh nods.*) But another part feels guilty about that, as if, by enjoying the freedom, you're criticizing Sarah.

JOSH: That's right! I never thought of it that way.

THERAPIST: Shall we get all these parts together to talk it over with you?

JOSH: With me?

THERAPIST: Yes. You're the one who's noticing them.

[*This is a simple way of calling the client's attention to the Self.*]

JOSH: Oh, right. Okay.

THERAPIST: Invite everyone who wants to talk to come to a table. Make it expandable.

JOSH: Yes.

THERAPIST: Do you see them?

JOSH: (*Laughs.*) One is a sloth. It's hanging from the back of a chair! Another is an old-fashioned schoolteacher with a ruler. He's severe! And then there's Tom and Huck lurking at the back. They won't sit down. And there's a bat flying in and out of a skylight above us.

THERAPIST: Lots of parts!

JOSH: Golly! I can feel the bat flying right in and out of the top of my head. What's it doing?

[*Parts can be in or out of the body.*]

THERAPIST: Ask.

JOSH: (*After a pause.*) Having fun. (*Another pause.*) Sarah was a practical person and very smart.

THERAPIST: And you?

JOSH: Our second son, Mark, is a dreamer. A lot like me. Sarah had to organize him. (*Sighs.*) Ah well. We all loved each other. (*Another pause.*) I have a part, I guess it's a part, that's worried I'll pick another practical woman.

THERAPIST: It's worried about a part of you who would choose another practical woman?

JOSH: (*Laughs.*) My mother told me I should make lots of money so I could hire a butler. (*Holds out his hands with an amused shrug.*)

THERAPIST: What does the worried part want for you instead of a practical partner?

JOSH'S PLAYFUL PART: I always wanted to be an inventor.

THERAPIST: Does anyone object?

JOSH: The schoolteacher wants to hit me with the ruler.

THERAPIST: No hitting. He can use words.

JOSH: He says it's out of the question.

THERAPIST: Being an inventor?

JOSH: Maybe. He's not sure.

THERAPIST: Does all this forbidding energy belong to you? Is he your part?

JOSH: He belongs to me, but his energy is a bit . . . borrowed.

THERAPIST: Does he need it?

JOSH: Oh, yes! He says I'd be a bad boy without it.

THERAPIST: Who says?

JOSH: My father. Besides, he's been doing this for so long. He says he can't change.

[*Protectors often respond negatively to the word* change.]

THERAPIST: We don't need him to change. He can just relax and try something new. What does he like to do?

[*I cancel the word* change—*which Josh used first—and skip to a hypothetical positive outcome that includes having choices.*]

JOSH: He doesn't know. Maybe nothing.

THERAPIST: So, if you could keep the dreamer part on track, would this teacher part be able to relax and do nothing?

JOSH: Maybe. He's very doubtful I can help.

THERAPIST: Does he see you?

JOSH: Yes.

THERAPIST: Does he know who you are?

JOSH: He thinks I'm the boy who's looking out the window at the back of the class.

THERAPIST: That's not you. Would he like to meet you? (*Josh nods.*) Ask him to look you in the eye and see who's there.

JOSH: He doesn't know me.

THERAPIST: What do you say?

JOSH: I'm the one who likes everyone. I like the dreamy boy. I like Tom and Huck. I even like you. (*A pause.*) He's thinking that over.

THERAPIST: How long has he had this job?

JOSH: Since I was little.

[*Parts come online at different times and have different developmental levels.*]

THERAPIST: What are the pros and cons of doing this job—for him?

JOSH: He thinks he needs to keep me in order, but other parts don't appreciate him.

[*Protectors want to help. Exiles want help.*]

THERAPIST: So, being this severe teacher guy has been kind of thankless.

JOSH: True. I'll thank him, though. He meant well.

THERAPIST: How about a vacation?

JOSH: He'd go for that.

THERAPIST: He could see how you do while he takes a break.

JOSH: Yes. (*A chortle.*) I'm afraid his class is planning to graduate whether he likes it or not. He looks upset, but I'm telling him everything will be okay.

Unlucky kids get to work instead of playing, lucky adults get to play at work. Psychologist Mihaly Csikszentmihalyi (2008) coined the term *flow* to describe an optimal state of being, involving full engagement in an activity that leads to a sense of mastery because it is challenging but not frustrating. Sarah, we can surmise, achieved flow by being organized. Josh, as we hear, got into flow when he gave free rein to his imagination.

EXERCISE

Unblending Practice for Between Sessions

This home practice exercise centers on noticing. The more you notice your parts, the more they will notice you.

- Choose a part to notice, and write down what you notice.
  - Do you see the part?
    - If so, how old is it?
    - What is it wearing?
    - What's around it?
  - What other senses are involved in your perception of the part?
    - Sound?
    - Smell?
    - Bodily sensations?
  - How do you feel toward it?
- If you have enough curiosity and your heart is open, tell the part:
  - *I see you. I am here.*
- Ask it:
  - *Would you like to see me?*
  - *How can I help you?*

Conclusion

We ask parts to unblend, but we're not asking them to go away, change what they feel, deny what they know, or disown their concerns. On the contrary, we're inviting them to speak directly, be seen, be heard, share what they know, state their case, make requests, voice their needs, and respect each other. We honor their strengths, celebrate their gifts, and affirm that the Self can only lead with their consent. In all these ways, the practice of unblending empowers parts, which is good. Parts cohabit with the Self willingly when they know that we know how important they are. And sometimes we want one of them to take over. If I'm playing tennis, squash, or chess, I want the part who knows the game to take over. If I'm baking a cake, I want a skilled baking part (or at least a part who wants to learn how to bake) to take over. If I am dancing, driving a car, gardening, teaching, skiing, skating, riding a horse, or writing a book, I want my internal experts (or learners) to take charge. And I want them to be in relationship with my Self all the while.

In IFS, we aim for the Self to stay in relationship with parts and be available as needed. We ask parts to unblend and make room for the Self. Once they do, we can use all of our various information systems (sensations, feelings, and thoughts) for communication and self-knowledge. But clients don't come to us fully engaged with unblended parts. They arrive in therapy suffering a lot of interference from their parts. Proactive protective parts (managers) inhibit the flow of energy and information internally and externally, reactive protectors (firefighters) interrupt the flow of energy and information, and exiled parts are out of the flow entirely. Inhibitions and interruptions (we call them *symptoms*) are safety strategies. In IFS we aim to show protectors that the client doesn't need those strategies anymore. We devote the first portion of therapy to their concerns and fears about not doing their jobs. Often, they fear feelings. In contrast, the client's Self welcomes feelings. When all parts are welcome and exiles return to their rightful place in the inner community, manager inhibitions can ease up, and so can firefighter disinhibitions. With enough inner balance, the mind is emotionally rich, complex, and lively—not without conflict, but with the means to negotiate conflict and practice cooperation.

CHAPTER 10

Navigate Obstacles to Unblending

I f the Self is in the lead and protectors are saying *yes*, we can move on to helping exiled parts. But if protectors are still saying *no*, I keep sessions flowing by following their lead closely. In this chapter I outline a typical script for the first portion of an IFS therapy. Then I offer some examples of how I stay in flow, keeping that script in mind but holding it lightly so I can help protectors who get anxious and run interference, or, if my expectations prove misguided, so I can be nimble with self-correction.

When Protectors Balk

Protectors are afraid of exiled feelings and block clients from taking the most direct route to retrieving their exiled parts. They see the client as a child who they expect to help rather than a capable adult who can help them. They are the worried anticipators, meticulous planners, bold actors, resolute warriors, and avenging angels who don't trust grown-ups. We therapists come to the project of therapy feeling confident of our good intentions and aiming to make sessions flow—then wary, worried protectors make them slow. When managers drag their feet and firefighters doggedly reject help, we have to be nimble, attentive, good humored, and willing to go off script.

   If protectors won't follow our lead (*Try something new!* we suggest), we have to follow them instead—moment by moment, question by question. Along the way we keep inviting them to be curious, and eventually, if all goes well, they are willing to jettison their overperformed old scripts.

This makes therapy, as I said in the last chapter, a lot like improv theatre. This chapter illustrates, through several cases with commentary, some ways of keeping a session going when protectors aren't cooperating. The box below outlines a decision tree for interviewing parts and includes some drop-down menus of questions and options in different situations.

Interviewing Parts: A Decision Tree with Questions and Options

- **Is this part a protector or an exile?**
  - To find out, ask: *Do you protect anyone?*
  - If the answer is yes, ask: *Whom do you protect?*
- **If the answer is no (because the part is an exile), ask for permission to help it.**
  - *Do we have permission to help this part now?*
    - If yes, proceed by asking the exile what it wants you to know. Take notes.
    - If no, ask the exile to unblend and be patient for a while longer. Promise to return. Take a note so you remember that promise.
- **When you are focusing on protectors:**
  - Invite them to a conference table.
  - Ask if they see you.
    - If no, ask if they are willing to see you.
    - If no, ask why not.
  - Once they are willing to see you, ask who needs your attention first.
  - What does this part want you to know? Take notes.

Empathy Throws a Curve Ball

Empathy, as we've discussed, has some possible pitfalls. These pitfalls are particularly relevant for adolescents as they play out a developmentally normal push–pull between identification with and differentiation from adult caretakers, siblings, and friends. Here is an example.

Serena and Her Emotional Twin

Serena was a cisgender, heterosexual, Lebanese Italian American college student at the end of her freshman year. She had a tumultuous friendship with another girl, and their friendship was breaking up for the third time as they headed off for the summer. I had been seeing Serena for over a year, and we both knew she had a very tender (probably preverbal) exile, but her protectors were absolutely unwilling to let her make contact with it because they feared being overwhelmed. She launched this session with complaints about her ex-best friend.

SERENA'S ANGRY PART: She called me a narcissist! She should talk.

THERAPIST: Oh?

SERENA'S ANGRY PART: It's me, me, me all the time with her. Do you like my new shoes? Don't you wish you had this car? Her father buys anything she wants.

THERAPIST: And what did you feel when she called you a narcissist?

[*Encouraging a U-turn.*]

SERENA'S ANGRY PART: Honestly, if she feels insecure and needs all of Daddy's gifts, it's not my problem.

THERAPIST: So, what did you feel when she called you a narcissist?

[*Still encouraging a U-turn.*]

SERENA'S ANGRY PART: Stabbed in the back.

THERAPIST: And then what did you feel?

SERENA'S ANGRY PART: Angry!

THERAPIST: What does the angry part say to you?

[*I know the angry part is blended, but I address Serena's Self to see if the angry part will unblend at least a little.*]

SERENA'S ANGRY PART: She should talk! If I say anything about myself, she starts *blah, blah, blah*—I have more, I have better, I am better.

[*The angry part does not unblend.*]

THERAPIST: And what does the stabbed part feel?

[*To help the angry part unblend, I ask about the part who feels hurt by her friend's behavior.*]

SERENA'S ANGRY PART: We were supposed to be like . . . friends. Same—same.

THERAPIST: You were?

SERENA'S ANGRY PART: Yes. It's not so easy to make friends in college. My parents are divorced, and so are hers. We like the same things. We were both lonely. I trusted her!

THERAPIST: When someone you trust hurts you, how do you treat yourself?

[*Again, I encourage a U-turn with the aim of focusing Serena on her reactive parts and locating her exile.*]

SERENA: What do you mean?

THERAPIST: Is it okay to notice that?

SERENA: I get mad at myself.

THERAPIST: You have a part who gets mad at you. What does it say?

SERENA: I warned you. Stupid!

THERAPIST: It criticizes you. What else do you notice?

SERENA: I get mad at the other person.

THERAPIST: So, one part criticizes you, and another part gets mad at her. We've been hearing from that part.

[*Naming the polarity.*]

SERENA: Yes.

THERAPIST: What else do you notice?

SERENA: I just end up hating on that person.

THERAPIST: So, the angry part keeps the spotlight. And what happens to the part who got hurt?

SERENA: It's gone.

THERAPIST: Well, I bet it's covered up, not gone. If you could help it, would the angry part need to be so angry?

[*I introduce the idea of helping the hurt part.*]

SERENA'S ANGRY PART: I'll never trust her again.

[*The angry part ignores me. As being angry seems safer than feeling hurt, it's not interested in unblending.*]

THERAPIST: I hear you. And we can help the hurt part.

[*I persist, and suggest a U-turn.*]

SERENA'S ANGRY PART: It's not my fault.

[*The angry part returns to its conflict with the critic.*]

THERAPIST: The other part says it is your fault.

[*Because the angry part will not unblend, I follow suit, and we go back to the protector polarity.*]

SERENA'S ANGRY PART: I'm supposed to be the goody-goody! I'm supposed to roll over just to have friends. I won't do it anymore!

THERAPIST: The critical part tells Serena to roll over if she wants friends? (*Serena nods.*) Would the critical part and the angry part let the Serena-who's-not-a-part mediate this disagreement?

[*Rather than speaking to the angry part again, I speak about Serena in the third person, name the polarity once again, and assert that Serena's Self can help.*]

SERENA'S ANGRY PART: Oh, I hate the goody-goody!

[*Once again, the angry part ignores me.*]

THERAPIST: Does it go away when you hate it?

[*I speak with the angry part directly.*]

SERENA'S ANGRY PART: No.

THERAPIST: If you can't make it go away, why not try something new? With Serena's help, you two could meet and talk. It wouldn't cost you anything, and I bet you'd find it interesting.

[*I emphasize the minimal risk involved with trying something new and offer a small carrot.*]

SERENA'S ANGRY PART: (*Annoyed.*) Oh, okay.

THERAPIST: Promise me one thing, though.

SERENA'S ANGRY PART: What?

THERAPIST: If you have any worries or complaints you'll speak right up. Don't hesitate. We want to know what you think and feel.

[*Inviting and encouraging wary protectors to speak up helps them calm down.*]

SERENA'S ANGRY PART: (*Placated.*) Okay.

Serena felt betrayed by her friend. I didn't know who had turned on whom first, but I suspected the process had become mutual at some point. The two young women had bonded due to the mutual empathy and identification of their lonely exiles and scared protectors, and then their protectors had needed to get some distance from all that sameness, closeness, and vulnerability. In this interaction, I first tried to get permission to help her exile, but the polarized parts who criticized her or her friend, respectively, could only focus on their disagreement. I wondered if Serena's protectors would unblend so she could connect with her exile. When that stalled, I kept the session in flow by sticking with the action and letting my agenda go. This was more productive and, in the end, her polarized protectors agreed to listen to each other.

Maladaptive Guilt at Work

Undeserved guilt, as we discussed, has no useful function. But vigilant social manager parts will promote guilt in the absence of a transgression for any number of reasons, including the fear of rousing a despairing exile if a relationship falters or, as in the following case, the belief that loyalty is essential.

● Sebastian's Good Turn Gets Punished

Sebastian was a 27-year-old, cisgender, heterosexual, Asian American graduate student. His caretaking part, who emulated his father, wouldn't let him set limits in a romantic relationship. As a result, he kept trying to rescue a girlfriend whose addictive process had undermined her ability to function or be in a relationship. His tenacious rescue efforts ended with her blaming him for her feelings of shamefulness (a problem that long predated their relationship) and her cannabis use.

SEBASTIAN'S CARETAKING PART: Marguerite said it was my fault that she was high all day. How could that be my fault? I would have done anything to help her.

THERAPIST: Sebastian, I hear you have a part who doesn't want you to be blamed for Marguerite's behavior.

SEBASTIAN'S CARETAKING PART: But she does blame me.

THERAPIST: Do any of your parts blame you?

[*Encouraging a U-turn.*]

SEBASTIAN'S CARETAKING PART: No. Why would they?

THERAPIST: Just checking. You've had a conflict. One part took care of Marguerite while another part got more and more angry.

[*I name his polarity.*]

SEBASTIAN'S CARETAKING PART: I kept trying and got frustrated, yes. I guess I could have left. But I knew I'd feel bad about giving up on her. So, what else could I do? And then she blamed me!

[*Sebastian names a different polarity, one between a persistent caretaker part and a part who was trying to avoid future guilt.*]

THERAPIST: Your angry part wanted to stop taking care of Marguerite, but the caretaking part said you would feel guilty if you stopped.

SEBASTIAN'S CARETAKING PART: Yes.

THERAPIST: No wonder you stuck it out so long.

SEBASTIAN'S CARETAKING PART: Yeah.

THERAPIST: How do you feel toward your caretaking part now, Sebastian?

SEBASTIAN: I appreciate him.

THERAPIST: Who does he protect?

SEBASTIAN: Everyone.

THERAPIST: Inside or out?

SEBASTIAN: Both.

THERAPIST: Is he worried about anyone in particular right now?

SEBASTIAN'S CARETAKING PART: Not so much. I'm fine.

[*The caretaking part is blended and has been throughout this conversation.*]

THERAPIST: Okay. Marguerite has been unkind to you. Do any of your parts need help with that?

[*Because the caretaking part doesn't believe he needs help, I'm looking for a target part to get some traction with an inner inquiry.*]

SEBASTIAN'S CARETAKING PART: I feel pretty good about myself.

[*The caretaking part sacrifices Sebastian's good sense, but he also helps Sebastian feel good about himself.*]

THERAPIST: Is the caretaker ready to relax, then?

SEBASTIAN'S CARETAKING PART: Yes. I did my best.

THERAPIST: How does it feel to say that?

SEBASTIAN: True. And sad.

THERAPIST: What was sad?

SEBASTIAN: The outcome.

THERAPIST: Your caretaking part, Sebastian, tried really hard but got slapped down for his efforts. Does he see you now? (*Sebastian nods.*) What does he need from you?

SEBASTIAN: To know that I'm a good guy.

THERAPIST: What's the most important thing about that?

SEBASTIAN: He wants to be like my father.

THERAPIST: Maybe he could use your help with that. He so wants you to be a good guy like your father that he couldn't let you make a sensible decision about a relationship that had become toxic. Do you see what I'm saying?

[*As Sebastian isn't registering any internal conflict over this part's penchant for self-sacrifice, I suggest paying attention to some costs.*]

SEBASTIAN'S CARETAKING PART: (*Reluctantly.*) Yes.

THERAPIST: How do you feel toward the caretaking part, Sebastian?

SEBASTIAN'S CARETAKING PART: I admire him.

[*This does not sound to me like Sebastian's Self.*]

THERAPIST: Yes, he's great. He has helped you in so many situations. But maybe he doesn't always want to have to work so hard. Would he like to meet you?

[*I want the caretaker to feel appreciated and to meet Sebastian's Self.*]

SEBASTIAN: He's okay with that.

Sebastian was trapped in a pattern of giving to a girlfriend who rejected his efforts and expressed no gratitude for his good intentions, and then he was shocked to discover how this arrangement opened him to blame. I checked on whether other parts were criticizing his caretaker. He said no. But the caretaker seemed blended, so I doubted we were actually hearing from other parts. On top of not admitting to any conflict with other parts, the caretaker had no ambivalence about its job. To maintain flow in the session, I had to let go of my expectation that Sebastian would discover internal conflict over his caretaking behavior. But his caretaker part did confess his motive for continuing to take care regardless of Sebastian's best interests, which was loyalty to his father. Because the part would not admit to any ambivalence or conflict with other parts, I decided I should just focus on getting him to unblend by introducing him to Sebastian's Self.

An Exile–Protector Relationship

The next vignette illustrates the relationship of an exile to a group of crushingly critical protectors. If we think protectors are going to be kind or caring, we might mistake a highly critical protector–exile relationship for a protector polarity. It's important to know the difference between protector–protector polarities and protector–exile relationships because in each case we have a different aim. If we're hearing from one protector about another protector, we have to learn about their conflict, ask who they protect, and then ask them both for permission to help their exile, which may or may not be the same part. But if we're negotiating with one protector about how it protects an exile, we just need to ask it for permission to help the exile. Here is an example of assessing and intervening in a protector–exile relationship.

● Etienne's Exile Needs Help

Etienne, a 50-year-old cisgender, heterosexual, married French Canadian immigrant to the United States, had some polarized protectors (the most dominant being a team of critics and a firefighter who looked at pornography), but he was currently focused on the relationship between some older boys who were protectors and a younger boy who was an exile. Etienne had grown up with four older brothers, and he had three grown sons. When he was 10 years old, his eldest brother died in a tractor accident. His mother became depressed and committed suicide a few years later. By the time of this session, he had been in therapy for 2 years.

ETIENNE: I have to get up in stages. I wake up shaking and sit in a chair in the bedroom for a while before I go downstairs.

THERAPIST: The shaking part is the one we talked to last week? (*Etienne nods.*) He doesn't protect anyone, right?

ETIENNE: Yes. And the older parts all think he ruins my life. They hate him.

THERAPIST: Would they hate him if you could help him?

ETIENNE: They say he's a hopeless embarrassment. They want him to go away—forever.

THERAPIST: Etienne, how do you feel toward them?

ETIENNE: (*Shakes his head and sighs.*) They're too harsh.

THERAPIST: Do they notice you?

ETIENNE: They do now.

THERAPIST: How do they respond?

ETIENNE: They get quiet and looked embarrassed.

THERAPIST: They're older boys, right? (*Etienne nods.*) How do you feel toward them?

ETIENNE: I want them to let me help him.

THERAPIST: Will they?

ETIENNE: They get so frustrated and angry.

THERAPIST: The harder they push, the worse he feels. Do they notice? (*Etienne nods.*) Would they be willing to try something new?

ETIENNE: Yeah, okay. It will be hard for them.

THERAPIST: What will be hard?

ETIENNE: They're used to doing this.

THERAPIST: But they don't do it because they're used to doing it. They do it because they're scared of his feelings. That reason would go away if they let you help him. Then they would be able to do whatever they want. What would they like to do?

ETIENNE: (*Shrugs.*) They don't know.

THERAPIST: They can think about that. What are they afraid would happen if they stopped harassing the boy?

ETIENNE: I'd be him.

THERAPIST: He would take over. (*Etienne nods.*) That wouldn't be good for anyone. But we could talk to him about not taking over.

ETIENNE: He doesn't like being controlled.

THERAPIST: Of course.

ETIENNE: He doesn't want anyone telling him what to do.

THERAPIST: How do you feel toward him?

ETIENNE: I love him.

THERAPIST: Does he hear you? (*Etienne nods.*) Would he like to be with you now?

ETIENNE: He just wants to be with me without being told what to do.

THERAPIST: Do that. Be with him and don't tell him what to do. Ask the older boys to trust you.

When Etienne looked inside, he found a quaking, shamed boy who was being persecuted by some older boys. As this boy didn't protect anyone else, he was an exile. The older boys were his protectors, not because they were kind—protectors can be kind or mean—but because their intent was protective. They wanted Etienne to forget the past and go forward despite all obstacles. They didn't want the boy's bewilderment, grief, dread, and shamefulness to stunt Etienne's life. Despite opposition from the older boys and the exile, I kept this session flowing in a couple of ways. First, I asked the older boys to notice Etienne's Self, and then I suggested that the exile could be with Etienne's Self rather than taking over. Hearing this suggestion as an attempt to control him, the exile balked at first. But because he did want to be with Etienne's Self, he was finally willing to dial his feelings down.

Is This Part a Protector or an Exile?

Once a client identifies a target part, I ask myself, *Is it a protector or an exile?*

- If it's a protector, is it interacting with a polarized protector or with an exile?
  - If it's interacting with a polarized protector, I ask both of them to sit down with the client's Self to talk.

This gives the client's Self a chance to ask questions that will illuminate their motives and concerns.

- *What's your job?*
- *Whom do you protect?*
- *What are you most worried about?*
- *What goals do you share?*
- *Would you be willing to let the Self help the part you both protect?*

As polarized protectors listen to each other, they realize that they share the overarching goal of safety and well-being. As they get to know the Self, they realize that they have a powerful ally who can do what they can't do, which is heal the exile and release them from onerous jobs.

Exile Overwhelm

The number one fear of protector parts is that they (and the body) will be overwhelmed with the panic, loneliness, and hopeless desperation of exiled parts who believe they are being shunned because they're unworthy of love. From an abandoned infant to the older child who is neglected, abused, or exploited, exiles are emotional landmines, and protectors do everything they can to avoid, contain, or defuse them. Here are a few examples.

● Marina's Ensorcelled Baby

Marina, a 25-year-old, gender-fluid, pansexual, partnered Cuban American graduate student, came to therapy because they were restless in their relationship and feared being bored in their chosen profession.

MARINA'S FIREFIGHTER: I'm wondering if I should try polyamory.

THERAPIST: Say more.

MARINA'S FIREFIGHTER: I'm restless. I always want to move on.

THERAPIST: Where do you notice that physically?

MARINA: In my chest, radiating out.

THERAPIST: How do you feel toward it?

MARINA'S FIREFIGHTER: In it.

THERAPIST: In it?

MARINA'S OBSERVING PART: Yes. And a little annoyed, a little curious.

THERAPIST: Does it notice you?

MARINA: It says, *Go! Hurry!*

THERAPIST: Still curious? (*Marina nods.*) What would happen if you stood still instead of going?

MARINA: (*A few beats.*) I'd die, maybe. I don't know.

THERAPIST: Ask.

MARINA: I'm seeing a dead child in a coffin with flowers on his chest. My mother took me to the funerals of families who drowned in the Mariel boat exodus from Cuba and told me never to forget. She is a right-wing Florida Republican, so, you know, we disagree about everything. I tell her she's enabling White supremacists and she tells me about dead children.

THERAPIST: Sounds productive.

MARINA: We started fighting when I was 12.

THERAPIST: Is the 12-year-old the one who wants you to go?

MARINA: The go part is in the 12-year-old but has many ages.

THERAPIST: Where does the go part want you to go?

MARINA: To get help.

THERAPIST: For what?

MARINA: I don't know. (*A pause.*) It says, *Can you raise the dead?*

THERAPIST: The boy in the coffin?

MARINA: I see a baby in a bright, sunny bubble. Its eyes are open, but it is very still. Time has stopped, but it's alive, not dead.

THERAPIST: Does the go part know the baby is alive?

MARINA: Thought it was dead, but sees the baby is okay. Someone put a spell on it.

THERAPIST: Why?

MARINA: So it would wake up in another time.

THERAPIST: When?

MARINA: (*A pause.*) Later. When things got better.

THERAPIST: Why?

MARINA: Mom was depressed.

THERAPIST: What does this ensorcelled baby need?

MARINA: To be held. I'll get it out of the bubble.

As we hear, one part put a spell on the baby because it was too needy for a mother with depression. But the go part thought the baby was dead and wanted someone to rescue it. Without a narrative context, which Marina was now getting, this sense of imperative felt like an uncomfortable but inborn, inevitable restlessness and dissatisfaction. As it turned out, it was neither inborn nor inevitable; it was that problem for protective parts, fear of emotional overwhelm.

Negotiate with the Exile to Prevent Emotional Overwhelm

- Exiled parts are desperate for help, but if protectors do not agree, we have to ask them to be patient. If an exile makes a jailbreak and overwhelms anyway, protectors become more distrustful, and we go back to square one with them.

- But if the exile agrees not to overwhelm, we can negotiate with its protectors, aiming to have them meet the client's Self and let the Self help the exile.

- Sometimes an exile says it would like to cooperate but doesn't know how to unblend. In this case, I do the following:
  - Point out that all parts know how to unblend:
    - *Are you always in the driver's seat?*
    - *When some other part steps up, what happens to you?*
    - *Would it help if the Sophie-who's-not-a-part (the client's Self) could be in charge and you could stay with her?*
    - *Let's practice that.* [Now I walk the exile through the dial exercise, speaking to it directly.]
      - *Imagine a dial, like a volume dial on a stereo, that goes from 1 to 10, with 10 being the most intense.*
      - *Put that dial in front of yourself.*
      - *The dial controls how much you share your feelings with Sophie (the client), not how much you feel. No one can control your feelings, but you can decide how much to share them.*
      - *Now I'm going to ask Sophie to tell you where she wants you to set the dial so she's not overwhelmed by your feelings and you can stay with her. After Sophie gives you the number, just let your feelings settle to that level and feel it together.*
    - *How is that?*
    - *Now that you can turn the dial down, do you want to stick around and watch as we negotiate with protectors to let the Sophie-who's-not-a-part help you? Or would you prefer to wait in a safe place and we'll come back for you?*

In this way, the exile can practice separating and being with the client's Self without launching into its story prematurely and overwhelming other parts.

An Angry Firefighter Part
Tries to Contain a Drug-Using Firefighter Part

Firefighter parts aim to bring relief from pain, and they've usually got plenty of options. They also pinch hit for each other. The last option (death) is, ironically, what even very destructive firefighters are trying to prevent.

Darby's Firefighter Parts Disagree

Darby, a 38-year-old, cisgender, heterosexual, Icelandic American, partnered male veteran of the American war in Afghanistan, had recently relapsed on fentanyl and had just been in an intensive outpatient treatment program. As he segued out of that program, he started individual psychotherapy.

DARBY'S ANGRY FIREFIGHTER: Let's get a few things straight from the start. I don't expect you to like me or my politics. Black Lives Matter is a terrorist organization that was created by looters and criminals, I hate towel heads with machine guns, and I voted for Donald Trump. So, can we just leave all that on the side?

[*Darby's White supremacist part takes the lead.*]

THERAPIST: Probably not. Want to hear why?

DARBY'S ANGRY FIREFIGHTER: Because you're liberal?

THERAPIST: I do have opinions about Donald Trump. I'll keep my parts out of your business, but we can't do this without including your parts.

[*I am aware that Darby is speaking from a part, but I don't say that to him yet. I use implicit direct access—that is, I speak to his blended part without saying, You are a part. However, I do take the opportunity to introduce parts language.*]

DARBY'S ANGRY FIREFIGHTER: What does that mean?

THERAPIST: As far as I'm concerned, we're all the same in the most essential ways. Our minds have subpersonalities, which I call parts. For example, today you started off speaking from an angry part. It seems to be angry because it expects me to judge you.

[*Rather than responding to his statements about differences, I assert our similarity.*]

DARBY'S ANGRY FIREFIGHTER: Okay.

THERAPIST: So, your angry part came here on the offensive.

DARBY'S ANGRY FIREFIGHTER: Yeah.

THERAPIST: Does it often chime in about politics?

DARBY'S ANGRY FIREFIGHTER: Yes.

THERAPIST: Would you be interested in getting to know it better?

DARBY'S ANGRY FIREFIGHTER: Okay.

THERAPIST: Before we do that, how do you feel toward it?

DARBY'S ANGRY FIREFIGHTER: I like it.

[*The part remains blended. I know I am speaking with it, but I still haven't made that explicit.*]

THERAPIST: What's the most important thing it does for you?

DARBY'S ANGRY FIREFIGHTER: Keeps me alive.

THERAPIST: Yes. Angry parts do that. Is it listening to us?

[*The angry part had been expecting judgment and criticism. Instead, I assert that it has an important role.*]

DARBY'S ANGRY FIREFIGHTER: (*Warily.*) Maybe.

THERAPIST: Can you see it?

DARBY'S ANGRY FIREFIGHTER: Yeah.

THERAPIST: Can we be curious about it?

DARBY'S ANGRY FIREFIGHTER: (*Irritably.*) I don't have to be curious. I know about it.

THERAPIST: Because you are the angry part. You keep Darby alive.

[*I see that the part won't unblend, so I switch to explicit direct access.*]

DARBY'S ANGRY FIREFIGHTER: Yeah.

THERAPIST: When did you start protecting him?

DARBY'S ANGRY FIREFIGHTER: A long time ago.

THERAPIST: What would happen if you stopped?

DARBY'S ANGRY FIREFIGHTER: (*A long pause.*) I won't.

[*I have no idea what Darby was thinking about during that pause, and I assume he wouldn't tell me at this point if I asked, so I don't.*]

THERAPIST: Okay. Here's what I understand so far. It's very important for you to stay on the job, and you don't approve of Darby coming to therapy, but you let him come anyway. Why?

DARBY'S ANGRY FIREFIGHTER: He's using again.

THERAPIST: And your concern about that is?

DARBY'S ANGRY FIREFIGHTER: I'm the one who keeps him alive.

THERAPIST: It could kill him. Okay. Here's what I propose—and it's completely up to you if we proceed this way. I propose that Darby, his using part, and you, his angry part, all get together and talk.

DARBY'S ANGRY FIREFIGHTER: Who's Darby?

THERAPIST: You tell me.

DARBY'S ANGRY FIREFIGHTER: He's a guy who can't control himself.

THERAPIST: That's the using part. I'm talking about a Darby-who's-not-a-part. Since the using part is doing a job, just like you, and won't stop until that job becomes unnecessary, I want you to meet with him and the using part. You see, we need to find out what the using part is worried about and who it protects.

DARBY'S ANGRY FIREFIGHTER: Okay.

In this example, an angry firefighter is polarized with a drug-using firefighter. The angry one, who expected me to shame him, went on the offensive immediately. I didn't take the bait, nor did I agree to *leave all that on the side* as the part demanded. Instead, I kept the session in flow by asking the angry part what it wanted (why did it allow the client to come to therapy?) and by pointing out that if we planned to influence the using part's behavior, we needed to understand its motives.

Firefighter Parts Don't Want to Be Controlled

When firefighter parts are afraid of being controlled, we can do the following to keep the session flowing: (1) Say, *I don't want to control you or take anything away from you, and I don't have the power to do that anyway*; (2) ask what would happen to the client if the part stopped doing what it does (this will reveal either a polarized protector—*they would work all the time*—or an exile—*they would feel too sad to function*); (3) validate their concerns by saying, *I don't want that outcome either*; and (4) offer to help. Here is an example.

● Ariana's Cutting Part Is Doing Something Important

Ariana was a 25-year-old, cisgender, lesbian Puerto Rican with a history of childhood neglect and a cutting part. She came to therapy after being left by her wife of 10 years.

THERAPIST: Is the cutting part willing to talk with you?

ARIANA'S CUTTING PART: It's not interested in stopping.

THERAPIST: I know. It keeps the suicide part from ramping up, which is important. We're not trying to control it or take anything away. But how do you feel toward it, Ariana?

ARIANA'S CUTTING PART: I understand.

THERAPIST: Tell it what you understand and see if you've got it right.

[*When a client says* I understand, *make sure that's true by having them tell the target part what they understand. The part will correct them if necessary.*]

ARIANA'S CUTTING PART: Yes. We agree.

THERAPIST: On what?

ARIANA'S CUTTING PART: This is okay.

THERAPIST: What would happen if it stopped cutting?

ARIANA'S CUTTING PART: I'd be overwhelmed.

THERAPIST: With?

ARIANA'S CUTTING PART: Bad feelings.

THERAPIST: We wouldn't want that.

ARIANA'S CUTTING PART: No.

THERAPIST: But what if we could help the part who feels bad?

[*Moving to the hypothetical.*]

ARIANA'S CUTTING PART: How?

THERAPIST: I'll show you how if everyone's willing. We can do it safely. We'll start by helping the part who feels bad to not overwhelm.

[*Don't get sidetracked with long explanations. Just assert that you are a skilled guide and get back to the point—in this case, that I can help Ariana negotiate emotional overwhelming with the exile.*]

ARIANA'S CUTTING PART: Why would the part who feels bad cooperate?

THERAPIST: Because we'll offer it exactly what it wants and needs in return for a little more patience. That's a good deal.

[*Schwartz (2017) calls this* being the hope merchant.]

ARIANA'S CUTTING PART: Okay.

THERAPIST: So can we talk with the part who feels bad?

ARIANA: The cutting part says yes, but it doesn't mean yes.

THERAPIST: Okay. How about if it goes first? We can start with it meeting you, the Ariana-who's-not-a-part.

ARIANA: It thinks this is all a big bother . . . but okay.

THERAPIST: I appreciate its willingness. Ask it to look you in the eye. Who does it see?

ARIANA: A weak, despairing person.

[*The cutting part does not see the Self.*]

THERAPIST: Ask the weak, despairing person to separate from you, and invite the cutting part to look again. Who does it see now?

ARIANA: A child.

THERAPIST: Ask the child to sit next to you so the cutting part can see you both. Then ask the cutting part to look you in the eye again. Who does it see now?

ARIANA: Me.

THERAPIST: How does it respond to you?

[*I'm wondering if this* me *is the client's Self.*]

ARIANA: It says, *What took you so long?*

[*The cutting part does see Ariana's Self.*]

THERAPIST: What do you say?

ARIANA: I wish I knew.

THERAPIST: Try this. You didn't mean to leave them alone, and now you're here. Will it let you help the child? (*Ariana nods.*) How do you feel toward the child?

ARIANA: She's so cute.

THERAPIST: Is she aware of you? Is she feeling you? (*Ariana nods.*) Is she willing to be with you instead of overwhelming you? (*Ariana nods.*)

With the exile cooperating, the client was now set to check in with protectors and get their permission to help this little girl. To keep this session flowing, I dodged a power struggle with Ariana's cutting part by asking it to meet Ariana's Self. The next example illustrates a polarity between two dangerous firefighter parts.

First and Foremost, Compassion

Protectors tie themselves in knots trying to answer the wrong question (*What makes me shameful?*). When the client's exiles feel loved, they get around to asking the right question, *What made you shame me?* The answer is less relevant (and possibly impossible to discern) than having the confidence to ask the question. For this, parts need support from the Self. If protectors aren't yet ready to meet the Self, they're getting ready. Our job is to be patient and persistent. We keep asking if they're ready. In this example, I persist, despite protector pushback.

● Nora Needs Compassion

Nora, a 41-year-old cisgender, heterosexual, Irish American, had been parentified in her large family of origin and had rebelled as a teenager. Her manager parts remained critical of her rebellious teenage firefighter part.

NORA'S MANAGER: I have six sisters and brothers. My mother worried most what other people thought about us. She beat my younger brother without mercy for wanting to wear my clothes and play with my toys because he was obviously gay. She moaned about my eyeglasses till I was 12 and then switched to my thighs. Now she's mystified that none of us are married, though one of my sisters is literally a rocket scientist and the other is a very successful lawyer. You get the picture, right?

THERAPIST: What was the worst thing about all that for you?

NORA'S MANAGER: I became a juvenile delinquent and ran off with an older man.

[*She names a firefighter part as the worst thing that happened to her after describing a very painful childhood.*]

THERAPIST: How do you feel toward the part who ran off?

NORA'S MANAGER: Embarrassed.

THERAPIST: Would the embarrassed part let you get to know her?

NORA'S MANAGER: I guess. But why should I?

THERAPIST: Because your other parts shun her, which leaves her all alone.

NORA: Okay.

THERAPIST: Does she notice you?

NORA: No.

THERAPIST: Would she like to meet you?

NORA: No.

THERAPIST: Why won't she meet you?

NORA'S CRITICAL MANAGER: I'm critical of her.

THERAPIST: How do you feel toward her right now?

NORA'S CRITICAL MANAGER: At the moment, kind of critical.

THERAPIST: Would it okay to be curious instead? (*Nora nods.*) Tell her that you are not the critic.

NORA: Well, okay. Then she thinks I'm boring.

THERAPIST: Who does she protect?

NORA: Herself, I guess. That's why she ran off.

[*I'm betting she also protects other parts, but I won't push that.*]

THERAPIST: Will she tell you more about herself?

NORA: She hated living in that house.

THERAPIST: Does she feel better now?

NORA: (*Considers.*) She's angry.

THERAPIST: Does that make sense to you, Nora?

NORA: Yes.

THERAPIST: Would she like someone to know more about her experience?

NORA: Yes.

THERAPIST: That would be you.

NORA: She sees me now.

THERAPIST: What does she want you to know?

Although the runaway would not say who she protected, we can surmise that her mother's chronic shaming was hurtful and that Nora had vulnerable parts who were exiled. I guessed the runaway was what we call an *exiled protector.* She protected an exile—or maybe the whole system—but was shunned internally as a liability, which often happens to angry parts. I kept this session in flow in a couple of ways. First, I rotated to the runaway as soon as Nora mentioned her, and, second, I kept asking the runaway to meet Nora's Self.

Protectors Summon Exactly What They Don't Want

It is a rule that protectors re-create and reinforce the very problem they wish to avoid or resolve. You can ponder why, but do keep it in mind because, whether you can explain it to your own satisfaction or not, it does happen. Here is an example.

● Callie's Protectors Hold Her Hostage

Callie was a cisgender, heterosexual, divorced, Scottish American woman in her mid-50s who had experienced food scarcity, neglect, verbal abuse, and violence in childhood, as well as verbal and physical abuse in her only marriage. In therapy, she complained about her neighbors, who were from Southeast Asia.

CALLIE'S FIREFIGHTER: Those people stink up the hall with their cooking, they're greasy, and their music sounds like a fingernail on a chalkboard.

THERAPIST: Shall we get to know the part who criticizes your neighbors?

[*Suggesting a U-turn.*]

CALLIE'S FIREFIGHTER: (*Grumbling.*) I know it! I am it. I'd move if I could.

[*The part is blended.*]

THERAPIST: When you think or talk about your neighbors, what do you notice inside?

[*Encouraging a U-turn.*]

CALLIE: My heart beats fast. When I hear that music and smell their food, I want to jump out of my skin.

THERAPIST: What do you feel when you're around people who are different from you, Callie?

CALLIE: (*Considers.*) Alone.

THERAPIST: They've got their own scene going, and it's not one you have experienced. You don't know how their food tastes or how to listen to their music. So, being near them makes you feel lonely. But you can't move, and they're not going away right now, so I suggest we help your lonely part—and the one who blames your neighbors for your loneliness.

[*Promoting a U-turn.*]

CALLIE: (*Glumly.*) It would be better if they moved.

THERAPIST: You can help the lonely part.

CALLIE: Nah. That's my life.

THERAPIST: I know it's been your experience. But you can help your lonely
    part.

[*Pressing for a U-turn.*]

Callie's exile felt chronically abandoned and lonely—and excluded
from the lively family scene next door. Her xenophobic, racist firefighter
part responded by blaming her neighbors, as if they were the cause of her
loneliness. Callie had grown up in a rough, insular neighborhood, and her
first response to difference was hostility rather than curiosity. As a result,
she missed out on the possibility that her neighbors might have been friendly,
in which case she could have enjoyed their proximity and felt less lonely,
illustrating that protective parts always get more of what they don't want.

I wanted her firefighter part to unblend so she would notice her inner
community. One part was shaming her neighbors to distract from her inner
critics, who were, of course, shaming her exile. I kept the session in flow by
guiding her to notice her vulnerability and by repeatedly asking her to do a
U-turn. Her protectors might have rebuffed me and just gone on complaining, or they might have gotten angry with me and tried to pick a fight. But
I knew Callie well and felt confident about handling those contingencies.
When externalizing firefighters are shaming other people, it's not good for
the client or therapist to be a nonprotecting bystander.

● Sinead's Managers Fear Disappointment

Here is another example of protectors recreating the problem they fear.
When Sinead, a 33-year-old, cisgender, bisexual Irish American who used
they/them pronouns, was 8 years old, they watched their mother get hit by
a car and die in the street. They grew up and became a war correspondent
for a number of years before taking a job back in the States right before the
pandemic of 2019. They sought therapy because they were feeling lonely
and believed they were drinking too much.

SINEAD: I'm an adventurous, cheerful person. I never look back. I guess I'm
    just lucky.

THERAPIST: What would happen if you did look back?

SINEAD: (*A long pause.*) Is that what I'm doing now?

THERAPIST: Would your adventurous, cheerful part be concerned about
    looking back?

SINEAD: I think so.

THERAPIST: What is its biggest worry?

SINEAD: That I can't handle it. (*A pause.*) That's ironic! Given what I've seen.

THERAPIST: Would it be willing to meet you, Sinead?

SINEAD: Who's me? It doesn't believe in me.

THERAPIST: No reason it should if it hasn't met you. But what has it got to lose?

SINEAD: What if I don't exist?

THERAPIST: You would have some disappointed parts?

SINEAD: There's no fairy godmother.

THERAPIST: Right. There's never been a fairy godmother. But maybe there is a part who could meet you and report back?

SINEAD: It might not be a good idea.

THERAPIST: Okay. What if the meeting happened far away where no one else had to watch or think about it?

SINEAD: Where?

THERAPIST: Where would be good?

SINEAD: A trillion light-years away at the edge of the universe.

THERAPIST: Would that be good?

SINEAD: Yeah.

THERAPIST: Who will go?

SINEAD: A gremlin. They're very private.

THERAPIST: Okay.

SINEAD: Gremlins don't answer to anyone.

THERAPIST: When you both get there, ask the gremlin to look you in the eye. (*A pause.*) Who does it see?

SINEAD: (*A long pause.*) A strong person. But am I reliable?

THERAPIST: You mean, the gremlin worries that you might disappear? (*Sinead nods.*) Has that happened?

SINEAD: I don't know, but it's concerned.

THERAPIST: Well, I guess it could happen. Let it know that you don't control other parts. They can take you out if they want to. But we can also ask them not to take you out and eventually, especially if you help parts who have been hurt, they'll probably be glad to stop taking you out.

SINEAD: It's thinking.

THERAPIST: Okay. Will it let you know? (*Sinead nods.*)

As the preceding interactions with Nora and Sinead illustrate, I keep sessions with protectors in flow by focusing on process rather than content. I want to hear who they protect and what they fear. But most of all, I want them to meet the client's Self, and I'm curious about anything that gets in the way. They can have many fears. They might, for example, be afraid of not being needed anymore once the Self is there. Or they might find the idea of having someone inside who can help too good to be true. Or, as with Sinead, they might fear bad consequences, including suicidality, if the Self were to prove unreliable. We have to address all their fears.

EXERCISE

Inner Theatre: Some Role-Play Options

Role plays can be useful any time in the first portion of therapy as we focus on protectors, but they come in particularly handy when clients have trouble noticing or engaging their parts internally and when they're stuck because their protectors are not willing to unblend. Here are several different kinds of role plays. If you think of other options, you can adjust the following templates.

Externalizing Parts

In this role play, the client externalizes their parts, as children routinely do. The therapist can use sand tray play with little figures and objects, or just put figures and objects on a table top. Pillows, scarves, drawings on paper plates, and so on can also be used to signify parts. If the client is reluctant to begin, try this:

THERAPIST: What needs your attention today?

CLIENT: Well, I'm not sleeping well.

THERAPIST: What do you notice?

CLIENT: I can't go to sleep because my mind is busy.

THERAPIST: So, you have a part who is busy thinking when it's time to go to sleep? (*Client nods.*) What does it think about?

CLIENT: Lists of worries, lists of woes.

THERAPIST: (*Picks up the figure of a little man in a suit.*) Could this guy be your worrier?

CLIENT: (*Considers.*) No. (*Picks up the figure of a bull ready to charge.*) I think this is more like it.

THERAPIST: Ah. (*Clears a space on the table for the bull.*) And what happens to everyone else when this one keeps you going at night?

And so on. In my experience, externalizing play is useful for anyone who finds going inside to be a challenge, which is particularly true of men who are not used to inspecting their feelings or revealing their thoughts to others.

Gestalt Chair Hopping

Another kind of role play involves the client moving around a room or between chairs and embodying different parts.

THERAPIST: As you sit or stand in different spots, invite the different parts who have something to say about this situation to embody—be the part and let it speak directly. You and I will listen and respond after we've heard from everyone.

CLIENT: Okay. What if the part doesn't usually speak?

THERAPIST: Great point. If it's a part who thinks but doesn't say anything, just say *These are thoughts* so we know the part isn't speaking out loud. If it's a part who moves, you can move. If it communicates by sensations, you can say *I'm reporting on sensations*. Would that work?

And so on. The idea is to help the part embody and unblend at the same time. This physical dialectic, the practice of being separate and together, isn't hard to do, but most parts (at least in Western culture) aren't aware of the possibility. Therefore, they need to practice.

The Therapist and Client Role Play

Another kind of role play consists of the client taking one role and the therapist taking another. As shown in the following, this can be done in a number of ways: (1) a conversation between two of the client's parts, (2) a conversation between one of the client's parts and the client's Self, (3) a conversation between a real person from the client's life and one of the client's parts, or (4) a conversation between a real person from the client's life and the client's Self. The client should choose who they want to be in the role play. And they might want to try switching between roles.

1. Two of the Client's Parts

THERAPIST: Which part do you want to play?

CLIENT: I'll be my sister and you be me.

THERAPIST: Okay. Where shall we start?

CLIENT: Start when I said *I want to go on Sunday.*

THERAPIST: Okay. I'll say that. Remind me what happened next?

CLIENT: She said *We agreed on Monday already. You always do this.*

[*The client goes on to describe the argument with her sister.*]

THERAPIST: Got it. If I forget something or don't have the right tone, stop and direct me. Okay? (*Client nods.*) Also, let's have a time-out plan. We'll both notice your parts as we go along, and either one of us can call time-out to check with them. Okay? (*Client nods.*) The aim here is to slow this down and see what happens inside you.

And so on. Again, we want the client to access their Self with its powers of observation while a blended part is in action. The more clients practice, the more easily they will be able to access this dialectic of consciousness in the real world later on.

2. One of the Client's Parts Talks with the Client's Self

This role play recapitulates what we do all the time in IFS therapy, but externalizes it. If a client's process is smooth and fast already, a role play could be a clunky interference. But some clients benefit from hearing their parts out loud and seeing them in action. The practice facilitates their access to dual consciousness, as mentioned earlier.

THERAPIST: Do you want to speak from Self and I'll be the angry part?

CLIENT: Okay.

THERAPIST: We've just heard from the angry part, so I'll repeat what it said. Ask all your parts to relax so you can listen and respond from Self as we try this little experiment.

CLIENT: Everyone's okay.

THERAPIST AS CLIENT'S PART: I'm so angry with my sister. She always has to have her way.

CLIENT AS SELF: And there's that part who stays on her good side by letting her have her way.

THERAPIST AS CLIENT'S PART: Yeah!

CLIENT AS SELF: I want to invite that part to join us.

THERAPIST AS CLIENT'S PART: I hate that part.

CLIENT AS SELF: I think you two might have more in common than you suspect.

And so on. The therapist can also move to another chair and role-play the client's appeasing part. Once this is complete, the client might want to try embodying one or both of the parts to see how that feels, too.

3. A Real Person from the Client's Life Talks with One Part of the Client

As in the preceding option, here the therapist takes one role and the client the other.

CLIENT: I'll be my sister and you be my angry part.

THERAPIST: Okay. Do you want to start? (Client nods.) Remember to stop and direct me if you want. You've given me some guidance, but I'm winging it here.

CLIENT: Okay. Ready?

THERAPIST: Yes.

CLIENT AS ANGRY PART: You always think you should get your way. You just think you're right all the time.

THERAPIST AS SISTER: I think you're projecting.

CLIENT AS ANGRY PART: I think you took advantage after the divorce because you could boss Dad around.

THERAPIST AS SISTER: Oh, really? I didn't see you making dinner or doing the laundry.

CLIENT AS ANGRY PART: No one asked you to take care of me!

[*The client is now sitting forward with clenched fists.*]

THERAPIST: (*Holding up a hand.*) Let's stop the music for a moment. What do you notice?

CLIENT: This part is really mad.

THERAPIST: How do you feel toward her?

CLIENT'S SELF: I get it. My sister was really bossy and I guess the worst was that she put me down a lot. She was angry, too.

THERAPIST: Let's take a break here and find the part who got hurt by your sister's anger. Would anyone object to that?

And so on. Note that as soon as the client names an exile (the part who was humiliated by her sister), I suggest attending to that part. I want the client's Self to connect with the exile and then come back to check on the angry part. This order is most likely to release both parts from their current dynamic.

4. The Client's Self Talks with a Real Person from the Client's Life

And one last option, the client's Self can talk with the therapist who is role-playing a real person.

THERAPIST: How about I'll be your sister and you help your parts unblend so you can talk with her from Self.

CLIENT: I think I need to help the angry part first.

THERAPIST: Okay.

CLIENT: She hates that appeasing part.

THERAPIST: How do you feel toward the appeasing part?

CLIENT: She actually has more spunk than I realized. She's young and kind of wily. She keeps a sharp eye out, and she knows when to put her tail between her legs to avoid getting smacked.

THERAPIST: Your sister hit you?

CLIENT: Oh, yeah. With kitchen implements or a kitchen towel. She was really good with the wet towel snap.

THERAPIST: What would she say to your sister?

CLIENT: *Yes.* That's what she said, but it's not what she did.

THERAPIST: And what would the angry part say to her?

CLIENT: *Why are you so weak?* And then the appeasing part says, *I'm not weak. I'm just smarter than you.*

THERAPIST: Would they be willing to call a truce and listen while you talk with your sister?

CLIENT: Okay.

THERAPIST: I'll be your sister. (*Shifting into role.*) We agreed on Monday. Why can't you just be consistent for once in your life?

CLIENT'S SELF: I know you remember us agreeing on Monday, but that's not what I remember.

THERAPIST AS SISTER: You're so selfish. You always mess things up.

CLIENT'S SELF: And I know you've felt that way since we were kids. You resented being told to take care of me. Of course you did. I understand that. I'd like to talk about all that, but right now we should probably figure out how to resolve our scheduling conflict.

THERAPIST AS SISTER: You can't come on Sunday.

CLIENT'S SELF: Okay. I believe you. I can come Monday, but I still have to leave on Tuesday.

THERAPIST AS SISTER: Well, that's too short.

CLIENT'S SELF: I agree.

THERAPIST AS SISTER: Well . . .

CLIENT'S SELF: Yes, too bad. Next time we have to be more careful to understand each other.

In this example, the client gets a more three-dimensional view of the appeasing part and is able to speak with her sister from Self, neither attacking nor appeasing. At the end of any role play, wrap up by recapitulating what you and the client have learned, thanking the participating parts, and asking what they need now from the client's Self. Take notes.

Conclusion

In therapy, all roads lead to Rome. We can start anywhere, but we end up at loss, vulnerability, guilt, shamefulness, and anger, and these feelings are what most psychological and behavioral symptoms aim to manage. In IFS therapy, we have many moments of choice, because many of the roads we might take would serve well enough. Experience and training give us mental drop-down menus for moments of choice, and when nothing on the IFS menu serves, we can borrow ideas from compatible treatment methods. We can also just stop to be curious. Whatever we do, the idea is to help the client get beyond shaming to compassion.

THE SECOND PORTION OF THERAPY

CHAPTER 11

Witness and Unburden

Most of us need, even crave, validation and acknowledgment. And when we've been shamed, being seen feels crucial. Clients who speak of being *obliterated, annihilated, exterminated,* or *erased* are saying that they were shamed for some feature of who they are—one of their parts. Moreover, when that part strove for acknowledgment and validation, it was repeatedly sacrificed inside by fearful protectors. Amnesia, denial, minimization, and so on all duplicate the message: *You don't matter, you shouldn't exist.* For most clients, feeling unlovable was the worst danger of their childhood. At least, that's what exiles say in therapy. Their Self listens and asks, *What do you want? What do you need?* The answer, which invariably involves connection and validation, is all that really matters. Here are a few examples.

● Esther the Egg

Esther was a 43-year-old cisgender, heterosexual, divorced, Trinidadian American woman who, by choice, had no children. Her mother had belonged to a rigidly patriarchal Christian sect as she was growing up and had been violent toward her and her younger sister if they broke rules or displeased anyone in a position of authority. Her father, an officer in the military who was often away, was also a strict disciplinarian. Esther had been in IFS therapy for 6 months.

ESTHER: These parts view me as a precariously balanced egg, which they're rolling along carefully. They're shocked to think that anyone else would be interested in keeping the egg from breaking—they thought this was their job. But they are very interested in the idea that we could keep it from falling or being broken.

THERAPIST: Is it okay for you to meet the egg?

ESTHER: First, they have to believe that the egg and I are different. They're beginning to see it's true.

THERAPIST: Does the egg talk to them?

ESTHER: They won't say.

THERAPIST: What does the egg need?

ESTHER: To be safe.

THERAPIST: Would they like to know more about you?

ESTHER: Yes. There are five or six of them.

THERAPIST: Ask them to look you in the eye and let you know who they see.

ESTHER: They're surprised again. And interested in getting my help. But first they have to watch me for a while.

THERAPIST: Do they know who I mean by *you*?

ESTHER: I am conveying it nonverbally. They like that I showed up.

● *A Month Later*

In the preceding session, the egg's protectors met Esther's Self for the first time. A month later, after they had been watching her closely, they agreed to stop rolling the egg around and let her touch it.

ESTHER: The egg shivers.

THERAPIST: What needs to happen?

ESTHER: It doesn't talk.

THERAPIST: So, what needs to happen?

ESTHER: I need them to let me put the egg in my heart. But they can't agree to that yet.

THERAPIST: What worries them?

ESTHER: They say, *What about us?*

THERAPIST: What do they need?

ESTHER: They don't want to be parted from the egg. I know what to do. My heart is a palace, so they can all live there. We'll put the egg on a silk pillow. (*After a long pause.*) Yes.

THERAPIST: Yes?

ESTHER: The egg is perfect.

THERAPIST: Do any of its guardians have burdens?

ESTHER: They've been afraid.

THERAPIST: What do they need?

ESTHER: None of us want fear in the palace. They will leave it in a safe.

THERAPIST: How does that feel to them?

ESTHER: It's a relief.

THERAPIST: Now what do they want to invite in?

ESTHER: Courage. Confidence.

THERAPIST: How does that feel?

ESTHER: Very good. They'll stay here. (*Pats her heart.*) With the egg.

In this session, we learned that the egg was perfect, which means it had been protected and was unharmed. So I asked if the protectors had burdens. Typically, protectors come to view their jobs as burdens after an exile has unburdened. But the main burden for these protectors was their fear for the egg, which they had tucked away. Their job was to make sure it didn't break. Now they could begin to relax.

● Elion the Worm

Elion was a 32-year-old, cisgender, heterosexual immigrant from Kosovo. He came to the United States with his family as a child and had some permanent hearing loss from the war. By the time of this interaction, he had gotten permission to help an exile who had a profound startle response that made other parts angry because it kept him up at night.

ELION: I see a long thing under the bed—my bed as a child. It says something garbled.

THERAPIST: Does it see you, Elion?

ELION: Not sure.

THERAPIST: How do you feel toward it?

ELION: Repulsed? But curious.

THERAPIST: Ask the parts who feel repulsed to let you handle this. (*Elion nods.*) Okay? (*Elion nods.*) Ask if anyone can translate the garbled message.

ELION: I'm getting, *It's hard to be a worm.* (*Becomes tearful.*)

THERAPIST: (*After a pause.*) Does the worm want your help?

ELION: I can't touch it.

THERAPIST: Because?

ELION: It doesn't want to be touched.

THERAPIST: What does it want?

ELION: It wants me to sit on the floor nearby.

THERAPIST: Do that. If it's stuck in the past, you can help.

ELION: It's deaf.

THERAPIST: From the explosions? (*Elion nods.*) What needs to happen?

ELION: I'm moving the house to a mountaintop in Montenegro where it's quiet. He wants his family to be in the house too. . . . They are.

THERAPIST: Good. Stay with him.

ELION: (*After a long silence.*) He felt like a worm.

THERAPIST: Does he see you? (*Elion nods.*) How does he respond?

ELION: (*Tearful again.*) He says, *Where were you?*

THERAPIST: (*After a long pause.*) What do you say?

ELION: I'm sorry.

THERAPIST: What does he need from you now?

ELION: Before the war, we went to the hot springs in the mountains. He wants to be there.

THERAPIST: Does he feel that you understand what happened to him? (*After a pause, Elion nods.*) Does he have burdens from that time? (*Elion nods.*) Is he ready to let them go?

ELION: His body shakes, his head hurts, he can't move. What does it mean to let that go?

THERAPIST: What would help him, Elion?

ELION: I'm putting him in the hot springs and getting in with him.

THERAPIST: What does he feel?

ELION: Hopeless.

THERAPIST: What is it like for him to have you there?

ELION: He likes it.

THERAPIST: What does he need from you?

ELION: Understanding. He wants me to stay.

THERAPIST: Is that okay with you?

ELION: I will stay.

THERAPIST: (*After another pause.*) How is his body?

ELION: He's starting to move in the water.

THERAPIST: If he's interested, we could try a little experiment to make him more comfortable. (*Elion nods.*) It's up to him, but he could put that hopelessness and all the shock in his nervous system into storage till he's ready to let it go—if he wants.

[*By now I guessed that this percussed, petrified boy would unburden gradually. But we could promote his healing by putting his burdens (fear, autonomic collapse, the sense of worthlessness) out of his body and into storage.*]

ELION: He's willing to try that.

THERAPIST: Have him choose a container that closes and is big enough to hold everything. (*Elion nods.*) He can put it all in. (*Elion nods.*) How does that feel?

ELION: Better.

THERAPIST: What will he need going forward?

[*Putting burdens in storage allows the part to take in what he needs without delay.*]

ELION: Quiet. Calm.

THERAPIST: Invite that. (*A pause.*) How does it feel?

ELION: Good.

THERAPIST: So, Elion, will you be able to check with him this week? Think carefully. It's best to be completely honest. If you're busy or other parts will interfere, we'll ask him to be patient in this safe place till we come back next week.

ELION: Yes. True. I'd like to say yes, but I don't know.

THERAPIST: That's fine. Let him know that you don't have a consensus yet about being available to him outside of therapy. Would he like to stay at the hot spring or in the cabin on the mountain?

ELION: At the hot spring.

THERAPIST: He can also leave those burdens in storage for the week if he wants. It's up to him.

Some exiles are ready to let burdens go in one session; others need more time. If they need more time, we can move burdens out of the body to storage for the time being. If the part is willing to use storage, it's likely to feel some immediate relief. It may leave its burdens in storage till the next session, or it may take them out. Because this is unpredictable, I say in advance that whatever happens is fine; the important thing is to notice the experiment.

● Gloria the Wicked

Gloria was a 49-year-old, divorced, Spanish American woman who had been raised in a conservative Catholic community and family. Although she had attended Catholic schools all the way through graduate school, she and her children left the church when she divorced her first husband. She discovered, however, that although she had taken herself out of the church, she had not taken the church out of her parts. In our previous session, Gloria had helped a grade school part escape an angry, shaming nun. In the process of unburdening, this part had released all the kids in the school, sent all the grown-ups off to rethink their attitude toward children, and blown up the building. In this session, Gloria reported on what happened after the session.

GLORIA: I felt great till I went to bed that night, and then I began to feel horribly anxious.

THERAPIST: There's more to discover.

GLORIA: I tried to check in with my parts on my own, but I couldn't. I just felt more anxious.

THERAPIST: What did you hear?

GLORIA: You're wicked! You will go to hell.

THERAPIST: Can you see the part who said that?

GLORIA: Parts. More than one. They're hidden behind a screen and they're singing that I will go to hell, like a church choir.

THERAPIST: Are they parts of you?

GLORIA: Some of their energy is not me.

THERAPIST: Ask if your parts are attached to the energy that isn't you.

GLORIA: Yes.

THERAPIST: Why?

GLORIA: They don't want to go to hell.

THERAPIST: Are you afraid of going to hell, Gloria?

GLORIA: No.

THERAPIST: How do they respond to that?

GLORIA: They think it's best to hedge our bet.

THERAPIST: Who do they protect?

GLORIA: (A pause.) The May Queen.

THERAPIST: Who is that?

GLORIA: Every spring the nuns choose a May Queen, and the mothers dress her in virginal white. I got picked. The day was hot. The nylon dress itched. The priest kept taking pictures of me. It was horrible.

THERAPIST: Would she like your help?

GLORIA: Yes.

THERAPIST: Before we help her, let's check with the parts who are afraid of going to hell. Do they see you?

GLORIA: Yes.

THERAPIST: How do they respond to you?

GLORIA: They don't think I know what I'm doing.

THERAPIST: What do you say?

GLORIA: Let's ask the Virgin Mary. (*A few beats.*) She asks what the May Queen wants.

THERAPIST: What does she want?

GLORIA: She wants to go to the Dairy Queen with Jesus and Mary.

THERAPIST: Does that work?

GLORIA: (*Chuckles.*) Yes. The Virgin Mary doesn't like vanilla.

THERAPIST: Will the scared parts go, too?

GLORIA: Reluctantly.

THERAPIST: Are they at the Dairy Queen?

GLORIA: It's a party!

THERAPIST: Does the May Queen have burdens from that day?

GLORIA: Yes.

THERAPIST: Is she ready to let them go?

GLORIA: Yes.

THERAPIST: How does she want to do that?

GLORIA: She's putting on blue jeans and setting a bonfire in the parking lot to burn the dress. (*A pause.*) She's throwing the priest's camera in, too. (*A pause.*) Everyone is dancing!

THERAPIST: How is that?

GLORIA: Can she let a feeling go?

THERAPIST: Of course. What feeling?

GLORIA: Humiliation.

THERAPIST: Perfect. Let me know when that's done. (*Gloria nods.*) What does she want to invite in?

GLORIA: Freedom.

THERAPIST: How are the scared parts doing?

GLORIA: They're scared.

THERAPIST: What do they need?

GLORIA: They're afraid of the priest.

THERAPIST: Is he one of your parts, Gloria?

GLORIA: How would I know?

THERAPIST: Ask.

GLORIA: He says no.

THERAPIST: Is anyone attached to having him in your system?

GLORIA: No.

THERAPIST: Well, he can't stay if he's not wanted. When everyone's ready, just send him out. He can go to his higher Self.

GLORIA: Okay. (*A pause.*) Okay. He's gone.

THERAPIST: How does that feel?

GLORIA: Better.

THERAPIST: How are the scared parts now?

GLORIA: Better.

THERAPIST: Now ask the scared parts if they're ready to let go of worrying about hell.

GLORIA: But what if he doesn't stay gone?

THERAPIST: What will you do if he doesn't stay gone?

GLORIA: I'll send him away again.

THERAPIST: Are the scared parts ready to join in? (*Gloria shakes her head no.*) Would they be willing to put their fear of hell in storage to see how that feels?

GLORIA: Yes, they can do that.

As Gloria's process illustrates, one exile's unburdening (the May Queen) can lead to more exiles wanting to unburden (the parts who were afraid of hell). If an intimidating person from the client's life shows up, we ask if anyone is attached to that person's presence. If so, we help that part. If not, the client can expel the person as Gloria expelled the voyeur priest.

● Olympia the Plague

Olympia was a gender-fluid, 24-year-old, single Greek American. They came to IFS therapy after being in and out of various kinds of therapy since childhood. Their parents had separated when they were in infancy, and they had grown up a single child with a fragile mother, who alternated between declaring that Olympia was her best friend and raging at her.

OLYMPIA: My mother had a lot of names for me. The storm. The cherry blossom. The plague.

THERAPIST: What do you make of that?

OLYMPIA: I was her mood. Cherry blossom was popular, but the storm could break through—not pretty. The plague . . . that was the real me. That's what Betty thought of having a child.

THERAPIST: Can we help that child?

OLYMPIA: Yes.

THERAPIST: Can you see the child?

OLYMPIA: She's under a blanket. But she says, *Don't touch!* The blanket is poison. She wants me to light a fire so she can get warm.

THERAPIST: (*A long pause.*) What's happening now?

OLYMPIA: I was standing in the wrong place. A hand moved me behind her so she could get closer to the fire without being seen.

THERAPIST: She's still under the blanket?

OLYMPIA: Yes.

THERAPIST: What needs to happen?

OLYMPIA: She says she's covered with sores and doesn't want to infect me.

THERAPIST: Would she like your help?

OLYMPIA: She wonders if I could stand to see her.

THERAPIST: What do you say?

OLYMPIA: I have an elixir for the poison, and we'll burn the blanket. (*A pause.*) So we burned the blanket and she drank the elixir.

THERAPIST: How is she doing now?

OLYMPIA: She's going to sleep on my lap in front of the fire.

THERAPIST: Does she have other burdens, Olympia?

OLYMPIA: I'll ask when she wakes up.

Because Olympia's protectors were ready to get help, this session went forward without a hitch, and the exile was able to unburden. That might not be all of her burdens; time would tell. Sometimes an unburdening happens sooner than one might expect; sometimes it takes a long time. In any case, don't let your expectations get in the way of meeting your client's needs. Stay experience-near.

> ### Shame after Unburdening: Two Levels of Protection in the Self-to-Part Relationship
>
> - We cannot promise clients that they will never be the object of shaming again.
> - Healing exiled parts does not confer immunity from feeling shameful.
> - We cannot promise that inner critics will retire for good. That alarm system is likely to persist, though the Self can help shaming parts turn the switch off.

So what are we offering for the long run? The Self-to-part relationship confers two levels of protection.

1. The Self disproves the message of shaming experiences by holding the part in relationship (or holding it literally).
2. The Self calms the whole protective system (it exists, but is less active) and heals the exile, giving everyone inside some needed peace.

If an inner critic activates again, just ask the usual questions:

● *What are you afraid would happen if you stopped doing this?*

And when you get shamed again, here's a good outcome:

● *I feel hurt.*
● *I find perspective, humor, and compassion.*
● *I challenge the message.*

● Miguel Has Existential Fear

Sometimes the only problem to solve is the feeling of being alone. Miguel, a 66-year-old, cisgender, heterosexual, married Colombian American father of one grown son, came to therapy because he felt unaccountably depressed after inheriting money from an aunt.

MIGUEL: I should be happy. I can retire now without worry.

THERAPIST: But?

MIGUEL: I'm . . . depressed, I guess.

THERAPIST: What does depressed mean, exactly?

MIGUEL: Maybe oppressed. I had nightmares when I was young, and they're back. I wake up feeling tired and uncomfortable.

THERAPIST: What do you make of the nightmares?

MIGUEL: They're about outer space and what it's like to die.

THERAPIST: What do you make of that?

MIGUEL: When I was a kid we had a privet hedge with a flat top on the side of our driveway. I would climb up there and lie on it whenever I felt bad about something. I'd look at the sky until my problem seemed infinitesimally small.

THERAPIST: And then?

MIGUEL: I'd feel better. But I started having nightmares.

THERAPIST: About what?

MIGUEL: Outer space. So I became an astrophysicist.

THERAPIST: Really?

MIGUEL: Yes.

THERAPIST: Did that help?

MIGUEL: (*Laughs.*) No! If you want to feel anxiety, look at the cosmos.

THERAPIST: Can we talk with the part who feels anxious?

MIGUEL: Yes.

THERAPIST: Where do you find him?

MIGUEL: In my chest.

THERAPIST: How do you feel toward him?

MIGUEL: Well, I know he's scared. What can I do?

THERAPIST: That part doesn't have to do anything. See if he will relax. (*Miguel nods.*) How do you feel toward him now?

MIGUEL: I'm concerned.

THERAPIST: What does he want you to know?

MIGUEL: (*After a pause.*) Space is vast and extremely cold. Why do we exist?

THERAPIST: What is it like for him to be with you, sharing these thoughts?

MIGUEL: He's glad I'm paying attention.

THERAPIST: What does he need from you?

MIGUEL: He needs me to understand.

THERAPIST: What?

MIGUEL: That he's always been aware of things other people don't notice.

THERAPIST: And what does he need from you?

MIGUEL: He likes being with me.

THERAPIST: What needs to happen?

MIGUEL: He just wants to stay with me.

THERAPIST: Does anyone object? (*Miguel shakes his head.*) Okay. One question for him. What does he believe about himself when other parts don't understand him?

MIGUEL: That he's too much.

Miguel discovered he could diminish emotional distress (the cause of which he does not name in this session) by focusing on the universe and making his feeling and the problem that caused it seem insignificant. This strategy, however, had the unlooked-for consequence of evoking existential terror, which a protective part subsequently addressed head on by becoming an astrophysicist. Nonetheless, the boy who first contemplated the

implications of being on a small planet in vast space developed the burden
of believing he was too much. He was grateful to be acknowledged.

Witnessing, Unburdening, and Time

Like water, subjective time has some unique qualities. Water is infinitely
malleable and takes the shape of any container; in response to the stimulus
of temperature, it freezes, flows, or expands and becomes a gas as its atoms
move even farther apart under the influence of heat. Similarly, subjective
time conforms to the individual mind; it can freeze (parts get stuck in the
past due to fear), flow in any direction (our most comfortable state), or
expand under the influence of emotional heat and hang in the ether (dissociation). In the psyche, time is a medium, not a linear experience. Parts
can move around in it, and their stories, like lilies in water, grow over time.
This is as it should be. Our understanding of who we are should grow. If a
part is frozen, we want to warm it up so it can get back into the flow of time.

EXERCISE

Rescript the Past, Rehearse the Future

If we superimpose internal experience on external experience, we run the risk
of looking either crazy or mendacious. If we undo reality in favor of a fantasy, we
end up feeling depleted and defeated. But if we hold both subjective and objec-
tive realities in mind, we access a generous, spacious reality that is greater than
the sum of the two realms. We want to remind our parts that subjective reality is
their prerogative. We cannot go backward or forward in time objectively, but they
can. We cannot shift shape at will, but they can.

Rescripting the Past

We aim to validate the client's experience of the past, but some parts hear the
idea of rescripting negatively. They think of denying, erasing, forgetting, and so
on. Therefore, I preface the suggestion that an exile can rescript its experience
with words along these lines: *What happened. We know that; we do not deny it.
We also know the part got stuck in that bad experience, so it continued inside. Now
the part can end the bad experience and get out of there. We can make whatever
needed to happen then happen now.*

      Here are the therapist's instructions for rescripting a traumatic event, which
can begin once the client has accessed their Self.

1. The therapist begins: *Ask the exile to take you to the place where it needs help.*
   [The therapist can come, too, if needed.]

2. The client describes a scene in which they were hurt. The therapist says: *Ask
   the higher Self of John* (the person who hurt the client) *to join John's misbehaving part so it can absorb and process what we're about to do.*

[This step aims to release parentified parts from their burden of responsibility for a dysfunctional caretaker.]

3. The therapist says: *Ask the exile what needs to happen.*

4. The therapist says: *Now ask the exile,* Do you want to do that or do you want my help?

   [The exile might instruct the client's Self to admonish the perpetrator or take some kind of action.]

5. When that is complete, the therapist says: *Ask the part if it's ready to leave that time or if it needs help in another situation.*

   [When the part is ready to leave the past, go on to the next step.]

6. Finally, the therapist says: *The part can come to be with you in the present or go somewhere else it prefers where you can visit. Where would it like to be?*

   [I say this because some clients have chaotic situations in the present and the exile would prefer a safer place until that's sorted out.]

   Once the exile has left the past, complete these steps:

1. Tell the client to ask if the part has burdens from that experience.

2. If the client asks what a burden is, explain that it is a belief or a stuck feeling that it would be having a negative effect on the part.

3. If the part identifies burdens, tell the client to ask if the part is ready to let them go.

4. If no, ask why and address that obstacle.

5. If yes, suggest that the part can let burdens go to one of the elements (light, earth, air, water, fire), or in any way it prefers.

6. After the part unburdens, suggest that it can now invite in any qualities it's been missing and ask where the part wants to be now.

7. Finally, check in with its protectors. Did they see the unburdening? Do they still need to do their jobs? If so, ask why. If not, what would they prefer?

Rehearse the Future with Managers

Fearful, scout parts are always rehearsing a negative future in order to inhibit exiles or firefighters. This exercise rehearses a desirable outcome instead and includes input from vulnerable parts as well as the R&R (rest and relaxation) fire-fighter team when they are less extreme.

   Start by going inside and asking for permission to practice an optimistic thought experiment regarding the future. If anyone objects, ask why and resolve that before continuing.

1. Once you have permission to do this thought experiment, locate an issue or concern that habitually activates your scouting managers (the parts who anticipate bad outcomes).

2. Invite your scouts to that expandable conference table and ask them to put

their job aside for the moment in favor of putting on creativity hats or just relaxing and listening. Then invite any other part to the table who would like to participate and pose these questions. Give everyone a turn to answer and write down what you hear.

- *Whom do you protect?*
- *If this issue/concern/problem were resolved in the best possible way for you, what would be different?*
- *What is your end goal?*
- *How can I help?*

Now, put all the relevant players on a stage (or in just the right setting) and rehearse that outcome (or those outcomes if there are competing options) in your mind's eye. Stop the action periodically to ask everyone—the players and their audience—for their observations.

- *What is it like to try something new?*
- *Do any concerns come up?*
- *If so, how can I help?*

Finally, set an intention for whatever needs to happen next and thank your parts for joining you.

Rehearse the Future with Exiles

Here is another way to use rehearsal. If an exile worries who it will be without its burdens, suggest trying it out. Here is the language.

1. *I hear that you experience this burden as integral to who you are. I know it's integral to your experience, but it's not who you are. Would you like to find out if I'm right?*
2. If the part says no, ask why and follow up.
3. If the part says yes: *Let's do a reversible little experiment. Choose a storage container with a lid or door that's big enough for the burden. Put it in. You can take it back out any time. If it's okay to leave it there for the moment, ask your parts how that feels. What do they notice?*

   Follow up on these observations.

   - If it felt good, ask them if they want to leave the burden in storage or let it go.
   - If it felt bad, ask why and follow that lead.
   - A parentified protector might, for example, fear that liberating the exile will hurt a dependent caretaker. An angry protector might not trust the Self to show up consistently and fear the exile being vulnerable.
4. If the exile is too worried to conduct this experiment, change your language and make it hypothetical (*If you were to . . .*).

When the experiment feels complete, thank everyone for allowing it or participating and set an intention for what needs to happen next.

Blue Babies

When I reached a certain level of proficiency and confidence with IFS— which is to say, when I was sufficiently able to be curious and help my parts get out of the way—clients started talking about preverbal parts. The first client saw a toddler standing in a crib, screaming and shaking the bars. She was floating above this scene at some distance. Behind the toddler, a frozen, blue baby lay on the mattress. It's not unusual for people to remember traumatic events as if they are looking down from the ceiling, often from the corner of the room. One of my clients had a team of two parts, *record* and *replay*, who would show her being sexually and physically assaulted at various times in her childhood and teenage years from above without any emotion or sound.* Others have described adult rape scenes from this perspective.

After I got one portrait of a blue baby, two other clients described an almost identical scene. An enraged toddler standing over a cold, neglected baby, demanding the client's attention. In a whirl of contradictions, one toddler said the baby was dead, wouldn't leave the crib without the baby, demanded that the client rescue the baby, and then got wildly jealous of the attention the client gave to the baby. The second client's toddler also expressed rage at the baby, but wouldn't accept help separately. Only one thing was different for this woman. She found herself standing right in front of the crib rather than floating above. The third client's toddler, who was rattling the bars of the crib and making guttural, screaming sounds, wept in frustration and complained that the baby ate its own poop. The toddler had a wet diaper, a dirty little t-shirt, and was cold. But, like the other two toddlers, she would not leave the crib without the baby. At the same time, she didn't believe the baby could be helped. She blamed it for

---

* When I asked the client to read this passage and decide if I could include it in the book, she replied that she was grateful for the opportunity to help others and asked me to provide a few more details about how her parts show up in IFS therapy. She was sexually assaulted and tortured, apparently from infancy, by a child sex ring in the military that included her father and other officers. Her mother colluded and groomed her. These are her observations (emphasis hers): "Most of my trauma 'flashbacks' are *videos*, from across the room, the ceiling, or through a doorway. I have learned to witness and retrieve two exiles: one silent (hostage) 'videographer' and the one being abused in the video. They have not met each other until I ask if they want to. Each event is held by *separate exiles* who live in the dark alone. It always unbalances my entire system when a new exile shares her event. It is shocking and totally unexpected every time. That is how secluded they are. If I am in my body, my parts say, 'I am behind the eyes,' which is a very different visual perspective than seeing rapes and abuse from across the room. Body sensations are held by *separate parts*, found and retrieved in separate sessions. Sense of smell, taste, auditory are held by *separate parts*, often as trailheads activated by a current external event."

making everyone go away. She wanted to kill it. Sometimes, she told the client, she put her hand over its dirty mouth until it turned blue.

These babies were literally blue. Meanwhile, other babies and toddlers who had reasons to be figuratively blue were also turning up in therapy sessions. Three clients, all women, had the experience of being shown images (perhaps by a witnessing part from the same time or an older part who had access to the memory and the infant's fear) of an infant being sexually assaulted either orally, digitally, or with such objects as a spoon and the neck of a bottle. Like some of the women with blue babies, these three all saw the scene from above. One woman had a clear view from above of a white-haired man doing things to a baby; another saw a dark-haired man from above and behind, and then saw closeups of his fingers and tongue assaulting the baby, who stared up at the ceiling; another saw her mother molesting a 1-year-old in the bathroom sink with her legs in the air. If the child moved, her head hit the faucet. Another woman saw a toddler walking between rows of cribs that held wrapped-up, silent babies in a room with tall, institutional windows that were darkened by shades but outlined in bright sun, so it was clearly daytime. Yet another found herself looking through a window at a baby in a crib. Nearby, a woman and a man were gesticulating and yelling at each other angrily.

What to make of all this? The idea that an adult's mind can watch a traumatic scene from outside the body and replay that image is strange. Stranger still is the idea that an infant's mind has this capacity. These clients were all adults with trauma histories who had spent years trying not to notice intrusive images, and, with one exception (the woman who saw the 1-year-old being assaulted in the bathroom sink was certain this had occurred), they had not taken the images literally. They could remember later traumas, sexual or otherwise, but had simply tried to ignore the intrusive images that involved a baby. We could do likewise. But we shouldn't forget that people who had safe childhoods aren't plagued with images like this. Nor, for that matter, are the majority of clients who did experience sexual trauma, neglect, or violence in childhood.

I'm left wondering what we don't yet understand about preverbal experience and the mind's capacities. In any case, the exiled babies who make an appearance in IFS therapy have simple needs. Sometimes they unburden as soon as they feel safe by vomiting something grotesque (worms, slime, and so on), and sometimes they defecate profusely. Sometimes they just need to be picked up. All of them need what babies need—to be held, comforted, warmed, and fed. Toddler parts need the same, but when they're protecting a baby, they also need the client's Self to take the baby off their hands.

Seal the Deal with Exiles

When protectors give permission to help an exile, focus on:

- The client's Self connecting with the exile.
- Repairing that relationship as needed.
- Witnessing the exile's experiences
- Asking about burdens.
- Facilitating unburdening whenever the part is ready.

Conclusion

In the first portion of therapy, described in Chapters 8, 9, and 10, protectors call the shots. In the second portion, described in this chapter, exiled parts take the stage. Exiles are not like protectors. They've been isolated. They don't have jobs. They're burdened with shamefulness. They want to be affirmed, validated, comforted, and loved. They want, in short, a witness,* but they don't all need to be witnessed in the same way. Some want to show the Self exactly what happened, and this will take more than one session. Those who are stuck in scary situations often need to rescript and complete those moments. Yet others are satisfied that the client understands their experience and want to get out of the past promptly.

Once the exile is in the present, we guide the client to ask two questions: *Does this part have burdens from that experience?* and *Is it ready to let the burdens go?* If an exile is ready to unburden, a gesture or rite involving the elements (light, earth, air, water, or fire)† is a popular option. On the other hand, some clients want to craft their own ceremony. The exile should decide. If it's not ready to unburden at the end of a session, I suggest that it store its burdens in a closed container between sessions and return to continue in the next session. If the exile does release its burdens, the client seals the deal by asking how it feels and suggesting: *Now that you've made space, what qualities do you need going forward? . . . Invite those in.*

If a burden returns after unburdening, it's an important (if generally unwelcome) piece of information about unfinished business. Patience,

---

*Marvin Gaye, and later the Rolling Stones, popularized the phrase *Can I get a witness?* in performances of a song written by Brian Holland, Lamont Dozier, and Eddie Holland. The saying, however, originated in African American churches, with the preacher asking for affirmation from the congregation.

†Michi Rose, an early collaborator in the development of IFS, introduced this Shamanist tradition of unburdening to the elements to the IFS unburdening process.

persistence, and inquiry are bywords for ultimate success in unburdening. That said, many unburdenings are lasting, easy, and straightforward. Exiles leave the past and shed constraints, extract false organs, clean off tar, wash away mud, discard backpacks of rocks, jettison the false identity of shamefulness, burn shaming beliefs, and get relief. Protectors watch and let go (sometimes incrementally) of their jobs. Once given the chance, the Self leads by following: *What do you feel? What do you want? And you? What do you need? How can I help?* Compassion, confidence, patience, persistence, kindness—these steer the hitherto hindered client back into the stream of life, which is a naturally unrelenting and creative process of transformation.

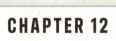

CHAPTER 12

Common Problems

So far we've looked at the following topics from the perspective of psychic multiplicity: *time* (external time is linear and inflexible, internal time is nonlinear and flexible) in Chapter 1 and in illustrations throughout all chapters; *shame* as a verb (shaming or shameful) in Chapters 1, 4, and 6; *guilt* (always prosocial, but not always beneficial) in Chapters 1 and 7; *protective intentions* (always positive for us; not always positive for others) in Chapters 1 and 3; *critics begetting rebels* in Chapters 1 and 4; the *goal of therapy* (self-validation and self-determination as a prerequisite for healthy relationships) in Chapter 2; *dual consciousness* (Self and parts) in Chapter 2; *variations on "no"* (psychic defenses) in Chapter 3; why therapy *takes time* (progress is a matter of willingness, not capacity) in Chapters 1, 3, and 4; *empathy* (empathy for pain is pain and evokes protective reactions) in Chapter 5; *parentification* (the child who got recruited into parenting their caretakers) in Chapter 7; and *parents* (who have parts and a Self, too) in Chapter 7. I've given examples that illustrate all of these assertions. In this chapter I do the same, with a few additional topics that are unavoidable in the professional life of a therapist, including anxiety, depression, major mental illness, forgiveness, endless grief, fear of death, and self-care. I also revisit racism.

Anxiety

A small jolt of anxiety is, as Freud said, a signal. *Get up! Study for that test! Don't forget to pick your kid up after the Aikido lesson.* And so on.

As Jerome Kagan (2010) pointed out, modern life rewards the anxious—up to a point. Too much anxiety is paralyzing. Kagan's research demonstrated the role of temperament in anxiety, but experience and the effects of experience on parts (the subject of this book) figure in as well. Let's consider, for example, the effects of shaming. If shaming hits a vulnerability in the recipient, especially a child, it stands a good chance of becoming an identity burden, a belief about one's personal worthlessness and unlovability. This state of being produces anxiety all around the recipient's internal system. Continuous-improvement critics are anxious to upgrade shameful qualities. Anticipatory scouts fear and plot to avoid the exile's exposure to more shaming. Dire thoughts, warnings, and physical paralysis (a.k.a. depression) suppresses unbearable anxiety about future shaming—or smothers rageful reactions to past shaming. And so on. The exile longs to be loved and fears being rejected. Reactive firefighter parts pinch hit for each other, counteracting the exile's anxious longings by self-soothing with substances, food, sex, dissociation, TV, meditation of the "spiritual bypass" variety (in which a protective part dissociates), online surfing, extreme exercising, and so on. In short, anxiety affects the whole internal system. Beyond temperament, anxiety signals the exile's underlying sense of worthlessness, which protectors fear. They may get frustrated with it or, alternatively, use it to control the person. Here are a couple of examples.

● **Bryce's Anxious Part**

Bryce, a 21-year-old, cisgender, bisexual, English Bahamian college student, came to therapy with me when her former therapist was retiring. She said she had been in therapy since she was 9 years old and liked having someone to talk to because it calmed her chronic anxiety.

BRYCE: I'm an anxious person.

THERAPIST: For how long have you been anxious?

BRYCE: Forever.

THERAPIST: How do you feel toward the anxiety?

BRYCE: I don't like it.

THERAPIST: Would it be okay to talk with it?

BRYCE: Okay.

THERAPIST: The parts who don't like it would have to relax and let you talk with it.

BRYCE: They don't like it.

THERAPIST: Okay. Put it in a room and you be outside the room for now. Who shows up in there?

BRYCE: It's a bent-over stick figure. Like *It's too much.*

THERAPIST: How do you feel toward it?

BRYCE: I wonder what happened.

THERAPIST: Is it okay with other parts if you go in the room to ask?

BRYCE: Yes.

THERAPIST: How does the part respond to you?

BRYCE: It doesn't notice me.

THERAPIST: Would it like to?

BRYCE: Now it's sidling over to the corner.

THERAPIST: How do you feel toward it?

BRYCE: I don't like it.

THERAPIST: Ask those parts to wait outside the room.

BRYCE: Okay.

THERAPIST: Now how do you feel toward it?

BRYCE: I wonder about it.

THERAPIST: What does it want you to know?

BRYCE: It's scared.

THERAPIST: How do you feel toward it now?

BRYCE: Concerned.

THERAPIST: Would it like your help?

BRYCE: Yes.

THERAPIST: What needs to happen?

BRYCE: (*Surprised.*) It wants to lean on me.

THERAPIST: How do you feel toward it now?

BRYCE: I'm helping it to lean on me.

THERAPIST: (*After a pause.*) How does that feel?

BRYCE: Good.

THERAPIST: What needs to happen?

BRYCE: It just needs to lean on me. It's unfolding.

THERAPIST: Is it your anxious part?

BRYCE: Yes. I feel this physically.

THERAPIST: What do you notice?

BRYCE: My jaw and shoulders are . . . looser.

Note that the part does not show or tell a story at this point; it wants connection with Bryce's Self. That connection launches a beneficial feedback loop physically. If Bryce stays with the part and continues to ask what it needs, she will eventually hear its story. An anxious temperament creates its own feedback loop and inflates worry into fear.

● Shira's Apocalyptic Spaceship Driver

We met Shira in Chapter 5 as we considered the effects of empathy. As a reminder, she was a 20-year-old, cisgender, heterosexual, Lithuanian Jewish American college student who came to therapy after a long history of anxiety, having participated in a variety of therapies. This was her first session with me.

SHIRA: I'm under a lot of pressure in school. I keep picking men who are critical of me and I have to break up, which is awful. I've tried family therapy, analytic therapy, and cognitive-behavioral therapy. I've taken psych classes. I know my father had a bad temper and picked on me. And I'm temperamentally anxious. So, I get all that.

THERAPIST: Why more therapy now?

SHIRA: Because an apocalyptic spaceship driver runs my life.

THERAPIST: Oh?

SHIRA: Yes. He runs my life.

THERAPIST: Does he have time to talk?

SHIRA: (*After a pause.*) He can't stop to chat, but he'll answer questions.

THERAPIST: Great.

SHIRA: This is weird. (*A pause.*) Isn't it?

THERAPIST: Yes. Is that okay?

● *Five Years Later*

Shira stayed in therapy with me past graduate school. Her temperament was still anxious, but she was, on the whole, happy. She and her lovely fiancé purchased a cozy house, she could usually calm her critics when they worried that she had made a mistake at work, and she was getting off other medications in preparation for getting pregnant. Life felt doable and negotiable. Just before getting married, she reminded me of our first session. *I didn't know what you were doing,* she said, *but I liked it.*

Clients like Shira who like IFS report feeling (over time) more spacious, relaxed, present, and engaged than they felt when they first sought help. They like noticing and interacting with their parts. They like having a way to intercede with internal conflicts. They like discovering that older, more capable parts exist and will step up to help younger parts feel better and relax. And, perhaps best of all, they discover that their psyche isn't intrinsically grim, gray, or boringly repetitive, even if anxiety or depression were making it feel that way. It's packed with motivated, interesting characters who have the power to annoy, frustrate, and frighten, but also to surprise and delight.

Depression

Many clients come to therapy having learned to use diagnostic terms to describe their problems. This is particularly true for the word *depression*, which covers a lot of territory. Depression is a physical as well as mental experience for most people. They feel slow, weighed down, and drained of energy. Either colors are muted or they don't see color at all. Cognitively, they lack interest. Emotionally, they feel disengaged, without desire or pleasure. Some people have a genetic predisposition for bipolar disorder and suffer severe mood swings. Accordingly, clients who use the word *depression* may be thinking of a protector who immobilizes the body to hobble an angry part or a suicide part. (Parenthetically, we know that the risk of suicide goes up when depression lifts in response to outside interventions such as medication and hospitalization.) Or they might be thinking of an exiled part who freezes and collapses in reaction to extreme inner (or outer) critics. On the other hand, they might be using the word *depression* to describe the sadness of a lonely exile. Ironically, exiling young parts causes them to feel hopeless, which, in turn, makes protectors think they're depressed when they're actually feeling sad and lonely. When someone uses the word *depressed*, therefore, I drill down for specifics. Here is an example.

● Tegan's Protective Depression

Tegan, a 69-year-old, Welsh American, cisgender, married lesbian mother of two grown children, came to therapy during a moderate bout of depression as she was on the verge of retiring from her long-time job as meteorologist for her state. She reported having had a severe depression in her early 20s for which she was hospitalized. She had taken selective serotonin reuptake inhibitor antidepressants since and had recently tried switching around with no notable effect. Although this was our first appointment, she had chosen IFS therapy and was versed in the idea of parts.

TEGAN: With my history of hospitalization, I'm scared of this depression.

THERAPIST: Tell me about it.

TEGAN: I used to have this happy image of life after retirement. But it's summer and I'm not even doing the things I usually love, like playing tennis and swimming.

THERAPIST: What do you do?

TEGAN: I go to work, come home, eat an edible, and watch TV with my wife.

THERAPIST: And what do you hear yourself thinking?

TEGAN: You're going to die.

THERAPIST: How do you feel toward the part who says that?

TEGAN'S WARNING PART: Hmm. . . . It's right?

[*The part is blended.*]

THERAPIST: But how do you feel toward it?

TEGAN'S WARNING PART: It seems to be telling me the facts.

[*Tegan has no ability at the moment to be in relationship with this part because it is too blended.*]

THERAPIST: Why now?

TEGAN'S WARNING PART: Because I'm thinking about retiring.

THERAPIST: How about I talk with it and you listen?

[*As the part won't unblend, I suggest speaking with it directly.*]

TEGAN'S WARNING PART: Okay.

THERAPIST: Are you there? (*Tegan nods.*) What would happen if you didn't remind Tegan that she's going to die?

TEGAN'S WARNING PART: She wouldn't make the most of the time she's got left.

THERAPIST: So you're trying to motivate her?

TEGAN'S WARNING PART: Yes.

THERAPIST: You're countering a part who somehow takes her motivation away?

TEGAN'S WARNING PART: Yes. She's depressed.

THERAPIST: Do you mean some other part restrains her?

TEGAN'S WARNING PART: I don't know.

THERAPIST: What do you notice?

TEGAN'S WARNING PART: She won't do things.

THERAPIST: Is it okay to find out more about that?

TEGAN'S WARNING PART: Yes.

THERAPIST: Okay, I'll talk with Tegan again. Are you there, Tegan?

TEGAN: Yes.

THERAPIST: Did you hear that? (*Tegan nods.*) Are you game to check with the depressed part? (*Tegan nods.*) Ask inside if anyone objects.

TEGAN: I don't hear anything.

THERAPIST: Think of a moment when you might want to do something but you don't actually do anything. (*Tegan nods.*) Where do you find that lack of interest or whatever it is in your body?

TEGAN: My chest.

THERAPIST: How do you feel toward it?

TEGAN: Puzzled.

THERAPIST: Would you like to understand? (*Tegan nods.*) Let it know. (*A pause.*) How does it respond?

TEGAN: It says, *I'm not who you think I am.*

THERAPIST: Do you know what that means?

TEGAN: No.

THERAPIST: Is it okay to ask who said that?

TEGAN: It's a girl.

THERAPIST: Is that a surprise?

TEGAN: Yes. I thought this was an older part. I was hospitalized for depression when I was 26 years old. I was supposed to marry a lovely man and I had just found out that I was pregnant—by accident. I didn't want to take any medication while pregnant, so I felt I had to have an abortion, which—my logic at the time—meant I had betrayed my husband-to-be and I had to break off the engagement. He didn't understand and, with hindsight, I didn't, either. But it seemed logical to me at the time. I just couldn't do it. So that was how I got out of marrying. I didn't know I was a lesbian until I met a woman 2 years later in graduate school.

THERAPIST: So, in parts language, you were about to go into a heterosexual marriage but, since you weren't yet consciously aware of being a lesbian and wouldn't save yourself in the more obvious way of saying no to the heterosexual option, a protective part saved you by making you severely depressed.

TEGAN: Yes. I think that is what happened. I also ended up getting an abortion, which was a huge relief.

THERAPIST: And now, facing the developmental milestone of retirement, you are experiencing another blue moment, though less so, which some of your parts are calling depression. Is this experience qualitatively the same as that severe depression in your twenties?

TEGAN: It feels similar, but not so extreme.

THERAPIST: What about that girl who said *I'm not who you think I am*?

TEGAN: Well, I don't know. That's not the depression.

THERAPIST: Okay. We'll come back to her. Ask the depression if it's trying to help you in some way.

TEGAN: Yes.

THERAPIST: What is it concerned about?

TEGAN: The sadness. It doesn't want me to retire. It thinks if I'm not busy, I'll feel too sad.

THERAPIST: If you could help the sad part, would it need you to keep working?

TEGAN: No. That would be okay. I think the sad part is the girl. But how can I help her?

THERAPIST: If you want, I can show you.

As we learn in this session, Tegan's depression warded off sadness. The sadness, we would learn later in her therapy, was an exiled 10-year-old who discovered, upon the death of her mother, that her mother was actually her grandmother, whereas her older sister was her biological mother, and her father (who died 2 years later) was actually her grandfather. Her biological father had been her biological teenage mother's boyfriend and had died in a car accident just before she was born. After her grandmother died, she went to live with a biological aunt (who until recently had been her sister), and she felt like an orphan who, to boot, had been fooled. Her feeling of being sad, lost, alone, and out of the loop had only been a backdrop to Tegan's later crisis of depression, which was instrumental and had saved her from a heterosexual marriage. But as the girl managed to get near the surface of Tegan's consciousness again when she was going to retire, protectors mistook her sadness for depression. This is not unusual for people with a history of severe depression.

● Griffin's Depression Team

Griffin was a 24-year-old, cisgender, single Chinese Canadian. His family was from Hong Kong, but he had Canadian citizenship and had gone to boarding school in Canada and stayed. He was now in graduate school in the United States. He started therapy as China was instituting martial law in Hong Kong, but he said he had a long history of feeling blue for several months at a time.

GRIFFIN'S MANAGER: I'm depressed.

THERAPIST: How do you know?

GRIFFIN'S MANAGER: I have no interest in things.

THERAPIST: What else do you notice?

GRIFFIN'S MANAGER: You mean like thoughts?

THERAPIST: Thoughts, beliefs, sensations, emotions, action urges.

GRIFFIN'S MANAGER: I think a lot about how it's too late. (*A pause.*) I feel heavy. Like someone put a weighted blanket over my head, and I can't get out from under.

THERAPIST: Is that one part or two?

GRIFFIN: (*Considers.*) Two. But they're allies.

THERAPIST: How do you feel toward them?

GRIFFIN: Smothered.

THERAPIST: Can we talk with them?

GRIFFIN: No. They don't recognize me.

THERAPIST: Okay if I talk and you listen? (*Griffin nods.*) So I want to talk with Griffin's depression team. Are you there? (*Griffin nods.*) What do you do for Griffin?

GRIFFIN'S DEPRESSION TEAM: We protect him.

THERAPIST: How old do you think he is?

GRIFFIN'S DEPRESSION TEAM: Twelve.

THERAPIST: There is a grown-up Griffin who could help the 12-year-old. A Griffin-who's-not-a-part. Want to meet him?

GRIFFIN'S DEPRESSION TEAM: No.

THERAPIST: How come?

GRIFFIN'S DEPRESSION TEAM: What about us?

THERAPIST: He would help you, too. We don't want to get rid of you. Though I realize other parts probably do. Is that right?

GRIFFIN'S DEPRESSION TEAM: Yes.

THERAPIST: Well, they just see what you do, not who you are. That would change if they met you.

GRIFFIN'S DEPRESSION TEAM: We don't trust you.

THERAPIST: Okay, fair enough. Tell us what you want for Griffin.

GRIFFIN'S DEPRESSION TEAM: He could get angry.

THERAPIST: And you don't want him to get angry?

GRIFFIN'S DEPRESSION TEAM: No. It's not safe. But if he's not angry, he feels helpless.

THERAPIST: And that's not good, either.

GRIFFIN'S DEPRESSION TEAM: No.

THERAPIST: What happens when he feels helpless?

GRIFFIN'S DEPRESSION TEAM: He wants to die.

THERAPIST: So you don't want him to feel angry or helpless?

GRIFFIN'S DEPRESSION TEAM: Right. We don't want him to feel at all.

THERAPIST: If the Griffin-who's-not-a-part could help the angry part and the helpless part, would you need him to be depressed?

GRIFFIN'S DEPRESSION TEAM: Probably not.

THERAPIST: I'm confident he can help those parts. But don't take my word. Meet the Griffin-who's-not-a-part and decide for yourself.

GRIFFIN'S DEPRESSION TEAM: What about the parts who try to get rid of us?

THERAPIST: Let's ask them what they want for Griffin.

GRIFFIN: They want me to be safe.

THERAPIST: Does the depression team argue with that?

GRIFFIN: No.

THERAPIST: So, ultimately, everyone has the same goal.

GRIFFIN: Yes, but they don't trust each other.

THERAPIST: Well, that makes sense because they don't agree on how to be safe. That's why they need your help.

When the client presents with a one-thing-leads-to-the-next cascade of reactivity (*We don't want him to feel angry but if he's not angry he feels hopeless and wants to die so we make him depressed*), don't let it interfere with your approach. You have the benefit of knowing two things that the client's parts don't yet understand. First, all protectors in one system want their person to be safe and feel lovable; second, connecting with the Self will immediately convince them of something they will not otherwise understand. This burning building has an exit.

Major Mental Illness

People who are diagnosed with bipolar and schizoaffective disorders say their mental timing is off; their minds go too fast or too slow. The psychotic mind, on the other hand, is swamped with distorted thoughts, and sometimes images, that block its ability to know what everyone else knows. It sees, hears, and believes in things that are not, by common consensus, there. When I was in training many years ago at a day treatment program for patients (as people in the program were called) with major mental illness, including schizophrenia, schizoaffective disorder, and bipolar disorder, I joined forces with two other trainees to offer a time-limited, open-topic talk therapy group, which was not the usual fare in this day program, but the staff were amenable. Anyone could sign up, and we had four takers. We simply opened the floor and they talked.

● Some Questions in Search of Answers

All four participants had been through psychotic, manic, or depressive episodes. One had removed his clothes while walking on the median strip of a thoroughfare in a big city. When the police arrived, he ran from them through traffic. And when they caught up, they threw him on the pavement, tasering and kicking him. Another patient had been hit by a car while walking on a largely empty highway at 3:00 A.M. She could not remember why she was there or how she survived. Another had been evicted from Section 8 housing after stuffing her mattress, blankets, and clothing against the baseboard heating units, which she heard criticizing her, and starting a fire. And the last person had lived for 3 years in the streets of a big city, unwilling to use even a blanket if it was offered by human hands after his parents, who had taken care of him well into his adult years, died in quick succession. All of these individuals were now on medication, which helped clear their thoughts but came with serious physical side effects. All could have reported very challenging childhoods, but they chose to focus on the more recent terrors and humiliations of being mentally ill.

The day program's knowledgeable staff members were surprised to hear that our participants were speaking about their experience with clarity and insight. They concluded that talking with students who would soon be leaving had been an unexpected opportunity. At the same time, I wasn't equipped to ask the questions that I would now ask, such as How do parts explain and relate to a malfunctioning brain? We know that protective parts will make use of physical malfunctions in pursuit of their goals, but do they understand that the brain is malfunctioning? Can they produce or amplify psychosis? Are they capable of speeding the brain up or slowing it down? I suspect they are, but much remains to be explored regarding psychic multiplicity and major mental illness.

Racism

From the perspective of this book, racism, misogyny, homophobia, transphobia, and all other rage-fueled, fear-based aggression constitutes the behavior of protectors who guard particularly fragile exiles. Although psychotherapy is not a social justice movement, people do come to therapy for the same reason they seek justice—to heal. Aggressive people, though less likely to ask for help and more likely to be mandated to get help, signal unmet emotional needs just as much as depressed, avoidant, or anxious people. In IFS, we welcome all parts. But how do we help clients who express or endorse offensive, provocative views and don't arrive in therapy believing they are a problem? As we've seen, the usual method of inquiry serves well with extreme protectors of all stripes.

More broadly, can this perspective on the internal system help us understand how the individual is shaped within larger systems? I'll take the identity group of White European Americans in the United States, my own cohort, as an example. This group, on the whole, struggles with the idea of guilt, rejects the idea of reparations, and continues to transgress, both passively and actively. Why? Here's one possible factor that relates to shame. As we've been discussing, the psyche is not monolithic. As a result, when a firefighter part transgresses, manager parts feel guilty. Out in the world, when an individual offends and is caught, they will, at least in theory, be charged, prosecuted, and assigned consequences. Similarly, when a group transgresses against another group, the surviving community may establish guidelines for repair that include an admission of guilt and opportunities for rehabilitation. This is the route South Africa and Rwanda took. With an accountability process, the aftermath of a transgression has an endpoint, and the prosecution can stand down. A community that can't concede the reality of past transgressions, however, denies itself the opportunity for internal as well as external repair, leaving the individual to the mercy of their own conscience—the court that never closes.

Short of admitting guilt and making reparations, a transgressing part will stand before internal prosecutors without relief. It may cause the person to withdraw socially, commit suicide, or, as we see in the White supremacy movement, fight back in a way that merits the label *sociopathic* because the individuals register no anxiety or regret about their aggression. An unrepentant transgressor avoids the voice of conscience by staying in motion. It will lie, protect material privileges, deny guilt or remorse, aggress, and maintain a sticky fealty to the past.

I'm proposing that the rage and aggression of the guilty who have not forged a road to repair aim, above all, to counter harsh internal judgments. When a conscienceless, anxiety-free, sociopathic individual (who doesn't have brain damage) is imprisoned, they become anxious and depressed (Vaillant, 1975). When we ward off inner shaming with cunning or rage and fail to register adaptive guilt and engage in reparations to settle the inner shaming and regain a place in the community, the emotional fallout can cascade down generations and cost a great deal more than being fair and settling debts, economic and otherwise.* As I've been arguing, we should not underestimate the power of internal shaming to motivate the antisocial behavior of firefighter parts. Whether or not you find this hypothesis possible or probable, you may find it useful (as I do) in calming your protectors so that you can feel compassion for offensive, blended

---

* A case in point: Robert McNamara's son, Craig, published a book in 2022 about his relationship with his father and with Rich Rusk, Dean Rusk's son, who committed suicide in 2018. The book is called *Because Our Fathers Lied: A Memoir of Truth and Family, From Vietnam to Today.*

firefighter parts even as they're being offensive. Compassion, by the way, holds people accountable for their firefighter parts far more effectively than shaming. Here is an example.

● Lance and the Rat Man

Lance was a 23-year-old, cisgender, heterosexual, English Spanish American man who grew up in a family that used overtly racist language and engaged in racist behavior. His bipolar father had been verbally and physically abusive toward him; his mother, who was largely out of the house working or socializing, had hired women to take care of him and his younger brother. In this session, 3 months into therapy, he was feeling comfortable enough to lob a transference test (as we discussed in Chapter 3) by being offensive.

LANCE: Are you Jewish? Because I don't want to be offensive.

THERAPIST: Why? Are you going to say something anti-Semitic?

LANCE: As my dear departed maternal grandmother would say, there are certainly good Hebrews. (*A pause.*) Joking. It's just that you people love Blacks and Asians, and I don't. Just saying.

THERAPIST: I thought your mother was a Sephardic Jew.

LANCE: I told you that? (*I nod.*) Well, yeah, she converted and ghosted her family. Not my problem.

[*It seems some other part of Lance had told me about his mother's ethnicity. I had had many other hints of dissociation between parts in his system.*]

THERAPIST: I assume there's something important in all this for you, Lance. What is it?

LANCE: I want to be able to be myself here. I'm not politically correct. Can you take it?

[*I hear this as a passive-into-active transference test. Lance is casting me in the role he had as a child when he faced aggressive adults. I assume his protectors want to see how I manage this behavior.*]

THERAPIST: If I can be straight with you? (*Lance nods.*) From my perspective, the important point in therapy is how you take what goes on in your head. When you say want to be able to be yourself, I'm guessing you mean you don't want to sanitize or censor your thoughts and feelings for my sake. Is that right? (*Lance nods.*) I agree. I don't want you to censor your parts.

LANCE: Which ones?

THERAPIST: Any of them. You have a part who says insulting things about Jewish, Black, and Asian people. And maybe people in other racial or ethnic categories, too. That is what goes on in your head. Is that right?

(*Lance nods.*) Well, this is the right place for what goes on in your head. For your angry, racist parts, and other parts, too.

LANCE: What other parts?

THERAPIST: You have lots of parts, Lance. Want to think of some very different parts?

LANCE: (*A pause.*) Okay.

THERAPIST: Think of someone you love.

LANCE: Meow—my cat. He's dead.

THERAPIST: Think of Meow. When did you get Meow?

LANCE: I was 5.

THERAPIST: Are the parts who loved Meow the same as the ones who insult other groups of people?

LANCE: No.

THERAPIST: Is the insulter a single part or a group?

LANCE: It's a group with a leader.

THERAPIST: Can you see them?

LANCE: There are five. The leader is rat man. He has the head of a rat.

THERAPIST: How do you feel toward him?

LANCE: His teeth are sharp. You know, people hunt rats. But he turns the tables. He hunts people.

THERAPIST: And given that, how do you feel toward him?

LANCE: I admire him. He's super ugly.

THERAPIST: What does he do for you, Lance?

LANCE: I don't know.

THERAPIST: Ask.

LANCE: (*After a pause.*) He protects me.

THERAPIST: From who? (*A long pause.*) Is it okay to say who?

LANCE: My father. That's what he says.

THERAPIST: How do you feel toward him now?

LANCE: He wasn't so bad.

THERAPIST: Your father?

LANCE: He's mentally ill. So what? He's rich. I never went hungry.

THERAPIST: How old does rat man think you are?

LANCE: He knows how old I am.

THERAPIST: When did he start protecting you?

LANCE: (*Smiles fondly.*) When he saw Meow couldn't do it.

THERAPIST: Can I ask him a question? (*Lance nods.*) What would happen if he didn't say mean things to you about Jews and Asians and Blacks?

LANCE: We're not going there.

THERAPIST: Okay. We won't go there until he agrees. Rat man is the boss. But would he like to get to know you better? He could see what you—the Lance-who's-not-a-part—have to offer.

LANCE: He's not impressed. But he's not running away.

As I've mentioned, shaming tends to aim at any (or any combination) of three major effects: restoring the shamer's damaged self-esteem by feeling bigger, stronger, and more important in comparison to someone who is being made to feel smaller, weaker, and less consequential; exerting control; or accruing power and profiting materially. Racist (or misogynist, transphobic, homophobic, ableist, etc.) parts can be physically violent, willfully provocative (as illustrated above), or insidiously shaming. But they are, in any case, firefighter parts who counter fear with belligerence and project exiled shamefulness onto others.

Forgiving

Protective parts have many reasons to be wary of forgiving. Would it lead to forgetting? There are parts who would like to forget. Would it cause vulnerability to the same insults in the future? Exiles are still vulnerable. Would it mean condoning a transgression? Some people in the client's environment may approve of the transgressor's behavior, and some parts will try to appease transgressors. Would it foreclose justice? Even when justice isn't coming, the longing for justice is a good source of energy and a powerful distraction from hopelessness and despair. The client's protectors don't know what we know, which is that forgiving doesn't mean giving up on justice, forgetting, condoning, or being more vulnerable—but they will learn. And the client's Self can choose to forgive without internal consensus. Parts don't want to be dismissed, denied, denigrated, or otherwise silenced. But if, like people, they are included and treated with respect, they don't always have to get their way. Here is an example.

● Eloise Survives Her Mother

Eloise was a 65-year-old, cisgender, heterosexual, divorced German French American. In childhood, Eloise was subjected to Munchausen syndrome by proxy—her mother had given her various inappropriate medications, starved her on the pretext that she was allergic to food, and taken her to numerous doctors who gave her mother attention.

ELOISE: I now see my mother in a long line of women for whom being female was practically fatal. Maybe some of them wanted children, but she didn't. She had ambition. She could tolerate a son because he enhanced her status, but a daughter was impossible. She hated me just like she hated being female.

THERAPIST: What's it like to see her that way?

ELOISE: I forgive her.

THERAPIST: All parts?

ELOISE: (*Laughs.*) Oh no! I have an angry 16-year-old who may always hate her.

THERAPIST: How does she feel about you forgiving your mother?

ELOISE: She says you can have your mother and I'll have mine.

THERAPIST: Does she protect another part?

ELOISE: She knows the little ones feel better now, but that won't stop her from hating Harriet.

THERAPIST: Seems like you two know each other well.

ELOISE: We do!

THERAPIST: She'll tell you what she needs?

ELOISE: She will.

From the bird's-eye view of her Self, Eloise saw her mother in context and understood what her parts should not take personally. Though her 16-year-old was not done with hating, Eloise got a good measure of peace from understanding that she was not responsible for her mother's rage and sadism.

Endless Grief

A popular old maxim says *time heals*, but the following example illustrates that time doesn't so much heal bereaved parts as it layers the psyche with more parts. We are able to thrive despite losses because, in addition to the Self, we have an ever-expanding pool of parts that appear in a developmental timeline throughout life. We are always multiplying.[*] Here is an example.

---

[*] For more on grief from an IFS perspective, see Derek Scott's chapter "Self-Led Grieving" in the book *Innovations and Elaborations in Internal Family Systems Therapy* (Sweezy & Ziskind, 2017).

● Annabelle's Grandmother

Annabelle, a 23-year-old, cisgender, lesbian, French-Dutch American, was 7 years old when her mother was first hospitalized for schizophrenia. She and her brother were left with their father, who molested Annabelle. After several months, her maternal grandmother intervened and took the children away. But when Annabelle was 10, her grandmother died. Annabelle and her brother returned to live with their father and mentally ill mother. Annabelle put a chain lock on her door and slept with a knife under her pillow. She came to therapy as a college student to manage the various aftereffects of this childhood.

ANNABELLE: I thought I would die when Grandma died. I couldn't imagine going on without her. I miss her intensely. She would sit next to me at night for as long as I wanted. I can smell her perfume when I go to sleep.

THERAPIST: Does the part who misses her know you?

ANNABELLE: It would seem rude to ask.

THERAPIST: Would it be okay to ask if that part needs anything?

ANNABELLE: She's sitting by my grandmother's grave.

THERAPIST: Waiting? (*Annabelle nods.*) For?

ANNABELLE: Her.

THERAPIST: Does she know that your grandmother died?

ANNABELLE: She knows.

THERAPIST: How do you feel toward her?

ANNABELLE: Sorry.

THERAPIST: Concern or pity?

ANNABELLE: Both.

THERAPIST: Can the part who pities her relax?

ANNABELLE: Sure.

THERAPIST: Does she notice you?

ANNABELLE: She looked up. (*A pause.*) She says *I'm real.*

THERAPIST: What does she need?

ANNABELLE: She wants me to sit with her. (*A pause.*) She says other parts don't understand.

THERAPIST: Do they harass her?

ANNABELLE: They want her to get over it.

THERAPIST: Why?

ANNABELLE: Well, to them this is all hearsay. They think she drags me down.

THERAPIST: So, for them, her feelings are too much? (*Annabelle nods.*) Would they let you help her? (*Annabelle nods.*) How do you feel toward her now?

ANNABELLE: Warmly.

THERAPIST: What does she want you to know?

ANNABELLE: She ignored them.

THERAPIST: Them?

ANNABELLE: The older parts. The ones who want her to go away.

THERAPIST: The older ones who never met your grandmother.

ANNABELLE: But they helped me survive. I'm grateful.

THERAPIST: Will they let you help the 10-year-old and younger parts who did know your grandmother?

ANNABELLE: Have at it. That's what they say.

Parts come online throughout our lives. In a practical way, ongoing development sequesters loss. Annabelle's grandmother died when she was 10, so parts who were 10 or younger felt bereft, but the parts who came online thereafter only knew her grandmother by reputation. While they witnessed younger parts grieving, some with more patience than others, they gradually asserted their interest in the present and future. And that, as Annabelle said, saved her life.

Fear of Death

Grief and fear of death can overlap, but they are not the same experience. When young children first encounter death, some are incurious about the implications, whereas others, who are more willing to tune in, are shocked and alarmed. When I run into young parts like this, who have been humming a grim tune about mortality in the background of a client's life, I am often struck by the existential nature of their fear. They were not speaking in metaphor about a different traumatic experience; they saw mortality and got scared. On the other hand, a child's fear of death can be a metaphor for the existential threat of disconnection from caretakers. Here is an example of the latter.

● Tess Doesn't Know Why She's Scared

Some clients have little internal narrative and no external knowledge of their early years. They have no parents, aunts, uncles, siblings, cousins, teachers, therapists, neighbors, friends of their parents, and so on to tell them about their childhood or their parents. They might have clues, such as strong feelings, intrusive thoughts, or memories in the form of physical sensations, snippets of visual imagery, or disconnected sounds. Tess, for example, was a 26-year-old, cisgender, heterosexual, Hungarian American who was adopted by a lesbian couple in Hungary when she was 8 months old. She came to therapy because she felt anxious on very cold days, was afraid of a bathtub full of water, and had intrusive thoughts about the people around her dying, especially her mothers.

THERAPIST: Is it all right to pay attention to those fears?

TESS: Don't say the temperature or talk about, you know.

THERAPIST: Okay. But can we talk to the part who is afraid?

TESS'S REPORTING PART: It doesn't talk.

THERAPIST: Can you see it?

TESS'S REPORTING PART: (*Shudders.*) It's a baby.

THERAPIST: Tess?

TESS'S DISTRACTING PART: (*A long pause.*) I'm running a 10K race this weekend, did I tell you?

THERAPIST: Okay. We don't have to go there. But can we ask inside about the intrusive thoughts? (*Tess shakes her head.*) No? (*Tess shakes her head again.*) Okay. I know some of your parts are in distress. Can we help?

TESS'S REPORTING PART: They don't think so.

THERAPIST: Who do they think you are?

TESS'S REPORTING PART: Too little.

THERAPIST: Them or you? (*Tess nods.*) Okay. Everyone's little. How do you feel toward them? (*No answer.*) I'll talk with them directly, and you listen. I want to talk with the part who tells Tess that the people around her are going to die. Are you there?

THE PART WHO WARNS TESS ABOUT PEOPLE DYING: Uhmm.

THERAPIST: Can I introduce you to Tess? Seems like you want to tell her something important. If you make just a little room for Tess inside, she can help.

TESS'S REPORTING PART: (*After a pause.*) It's gone.

THERAPIST: What happened?

TESS'S DISSOCIATIVE PART: I don't know.

THERAPIST: Did the part decide to leave, or did the dissociative part come in?

TESS'S DISSOCIATIVE PART: I don't know.

THERAPIST: Okay. That's fine. We'll wait to hear from anyone who wants to communicate with you. A part could be really young, but it could still meet you and get help.

As this session illustrates, when blended protectors are too scared of being overwhelmed by an exiled part to cooperate, the client has little or no traction to access their Self, and the therapist's Self has little authority to help the client's Self get better traction. In these cases, therapy requires long-term patience and willingness on the client's part to engage rather than avoid, which can be a big challenge. Therapists who specialize in dissociative disorders have a kitbag of strategies for helping protective parts who are too fearful to unblend. For an IFS tailored version of such strategies, see Joanne Twombly's 2022 book, *Trauma and Dissociation Informed Internal Family Systems.**

Brushing Teeth

Personal maintenance, known in the mental health and medical world as *activities of daily living,* or ADLs, can feel like an overwhelming challenge for people who experienced childhood trauma, particularly neglect. Thinking in terms of parts, the client who struggles with ADLs often has some young parts who feel yawningly needy. For them, self-care behaviors only serve to evoke neediness and grief about feeling unloved. If protective parts decide that recruiting outside help is the best way to address these problems, the result is an adult who cannot use adult resources to perform even basic self-care measures. Here is an example.

● Maeve Doesn't Want To

Maeve was a 32-year-old, cisgender, heterosexual, partnered mixed-race adoptee. Her adoptive parents were White European Americans. Her adoptive father died when she was 7, and her adoptive mother, a controlling, rageful woman, combined purposeful neglect with verbal and physical abuse.

MAEVE'S REPORTING PART: One part of me is like Cinderella. Another part doesn't want Cinderella to work anymore and tells her that she doesn't have to do anything, including brushing her teeth, because there's

---

* That said, I'm optimistic that new medication options like MDMA, psychedelics, ketamine, or neurofeedback have the potential to make therapy more doable for people with this kind of internal experience.

never been anything in it for her. Another part feels guilty about that. They fight all the time, so I get something done occasionally, but my teeth are falling apart.

THERAPIST: Who needs your attention first?

MAEVE'S REPORTING PART: None of them want my attention. You know why?

THERAPIST: Why?

MAEVE'S REPORTING PART: They don't believe I exist. And I agree with them.

THERAPIST: Who do they think you are?

MAEVE'S REPORTING PART: Someone who has never helped them and can't.

THERAPIST: So they see you as a helpless part. Would the helpless part be willing to move over and make room for you?

MAEVE'S REPORTING PART: They think you're dangerous.

THERAPIST: Why?

MAEVE'S REPORTING PART: You're selling the same old snake oil.

THERAPIST: Which is?

MAEVE'S REPORTING PART: I have to take care of myself.

THERAPIST: For the record, I want you to take care of them, which won't preclude others taking care of you, too. But they have to let you in, and they don't know you yet. That's why I want to introduce you. (*Silence.*) What was the worst thing about not having anyone to take care of you?

[*I made my case, but my words came from a defensive part and got no response. Hearing myself and realizing my mistake, I pivoted to curiosity.*]

MAEVE: I was alone.

THERAPIST: And what was the worst thing about being alone?

MAEVE: Imagine being immortal and alone on a rock in the middle of the ocean with no hope of rescue. You exist, but you don't exist.

THERAPIST: And if you brush your teeth?

MAEVE: It's just a reminder that you don't exist.

If protective parts are hostile or just implacable, you can always be curious. Curiosity will help your parts be patient and interested in whatever happens. The trick is knowing when to revisit the idea that the Self exists. As long as the client's protectors seem rigid, humorless, or brittle, I ask questions and listen. But if they can tolerate some humor and I feel we're connecting well enough, then I'll keep inviting them to meet the client's Self. If they're not ready, I'll back off. But then I circle around to the question again: *Are you willing to meet the Self now?* As with Tess, new medications like MDMA and psilocybin may prove helpful for someone like Maeve.

Conclusion

When we inquire inside, we repeatedly discover that our parts mean well for someone. So even if our behaviors have had a bad effect on everyone, we can stop accepting shaming. We're not perfect, but we are good. We're also completely capable of behaving badly. In fact, we're guaranteed to behave badly at times. When we do, we need to make repairs. We can own, understand, and take responsibility for our needs and our behaviors. Nonetheless, by embracing the plural mind, we set the stage for safe enough intimacy and our full potential for ethical relating.

CHAPTER 13

Take a Tip to Avoid Pitfalls

Of course, this book doesn't cover all the populations or the full range of symptom clusters that a therapist might come across in psychotherapy. But I've learned the ins and outs of applying the IFS approach with a wide range of presenting problems, and I have a few more pragmatic pointers for you in this chapter. Some are broadly applicable; some will only be relevant for certain people. In any case, I learned it all from my own parts or those of my clients.

Tips on Unblending

Unblending Is the Whole Ball Game

Protectors, as we've seen, are fearful and reluctant. We want them to unblend; to make that happen, we have to address their concerns. We listen, coax, and explain; we are patient and playful. Although exiles may need the Self to apologize for its long absence, they're ready to be seen and known as soon as protectors permit. Because witnessing reverses their banishment and undoes the judgments of shaming, it heals.

Age Matters

We have different expectations for children depending on their age. We're charmed when a toddler takes a tiny chair out of a dollhouse and sits on it. We're annoyed (or worried) if a 5-year-old does the same thing. Our intuitive sense of what is developmentally appropriate helps us interact with parts. For this reason, I like to ask about a part's age. Here are a few suggestions for helping parts of different ages to unblend.

Preverbal Babies, Birth to 1 Year Old

Get permission for the client's Self to hold the baby.

- Don't be fooled by reports that the baby is dead; let parts who guard it know that it's alive and can revive. Introduce them to the client's Self. If that goes smoothly, just ask the client's Self what needs to happen next.
- You may hear about what some clients call *video footage* (images from above) of an adult transgressing on a baby—if you are concerned that any of your parts could react strongly to graphic information about an infant being molested, prepare them by asking what they might need if this were to happen. For example, they might want to go into a sound-proof room and listen to music or go off somewhere else. Your parts are not obliged to witness disturbing scenes.

Toddlers, 1–3 Years Old

If a toddler part protects a baby, think of the toddler as an exiled protector. It stayed to protect the baby, but it feels trapped and furious, blames the baby, and desperately wants attention for itself. Don't ask it to step aside; include it every step of the way with equal attention. For the purposes of treatment, consider the baby and the toddler to be one unit until (if) the toddler chooses to peel off and go play.

- Don't ask toddler parts who are protecting babies to step back; they need attention, too.
- Listen.
- Validate.
- Reassure the toddler that the baby isn't dead, even if it's cold and blue.
- Ask the toddler for permission to take care of the baby.
- Ask the toddler what it needs before helping the baby.
- Once the toddler is willing, pick the baby up and take it (and the toddler) to a safe, comfortable place—the present, if that suits.
- Offer cozy blankets, food, and so on.
- The client may need to be creative about giving attention to the toddler and the baby at the same time—maybe by picking them up together, sharing the lap, or whatever arrangement the toddler prefers.
  - If clients have access to their Self, they will do all this without prompting. But if the toddler feels left out, a little guidance on

including it with the baby usually suffices. If that isn't working, check for interfering parts and listen to their concerns.

- Ask what the baby and toddler need in order to let go of their burdens.
  - Often babies shed their burdens over time by staying with the Self.
  - Toddlers may need some witnessing and may be more specific or even playful about letting burdens go. On the other hand, a toddler may let its burdens go spontaneously when it feels safe in connection with the Self.

Grade School, 7-12 Years Old

Protective parts who are 7–8 years old take a leap forward in their sense of responsibility for others and can be remarkably persistent about it, even when the client has some access to their Self.

Middle School, 12-14 Years Old

Between bodily and hormonal changes, this group undergoes a transition that makes them newly vulnerable. Substances, when they have access, are a great soother of shamefulness, fears of shaming, and reactivity in the case of actual shaming.

High School, 14-18 Years Old

As teenagers grow into some physical prowess and are headed toward greater independence, their angry, rebellious parts have the power to act when they feel wronged or endangered. Clients often report that they fought back against aggressive caretakers at this age and that conflicts that were hitherto emotional and verbal became violent.

Young Adult

It's not unusual for college students and young working adults to feel lost or overwhelmed, to become sexually promiscuous, to use substances to excess, to feel anxious, or to get depressed. Think of manager parts working overtime to discern how to fit in or succeed. Managers in this age group work hard. They look for inclusion, career success, and love. They work hard to anticipate and buffer potentially shaming social and sexual interactions. In response, firefighters distract, soothing nerves with substances and greasing the works for compliance in, for example, sexual encounters that are uncomfortable but offer the promise of comfort to lonely exiles. Between ambition and distraction, this age group often needs persistent attention to manager–firefighter polarities.

Age Matters, in Sum

Your intuitive understanding of age-appropriate behavior will help you navigate stuck moments with clients. You know that the terrified 3-year-old who can't speak, the scared 8-year-old who worries and scolds, and the fearful 18-year-old who drinks are all responding to their fears in an age-dependent way. When you talk with protectors about quitting their jobs and doing something different, try using open-ended language, such as *What might interest you now? What's next for you? What are you drawn to?* or *What calls to you?* so the part can make an age-appropriate choice. Often, they just want to go play.

Psychic Development Builds on Loss

Our offspring replace us just as we replace our ancestors. Along the way, we lose people, relationships, objects, projects, and expectations. Our parts differ from each other. They may have had different experiences with the same people. They may have known different people. They've lived in different times in different ways with different capacities. Each part has its own losses. Accordingly, they have singular needs and unique tales to tell. In this way, the psyche is as layered by the perspectives and ages of its residents as any community. Ironically, we can get more peace of mind, balance, and internal harmony by welcoming all parts than by trying to impose sameness or exiling those who can't (or won't) conform. The process of losing and replacing as we move through time is unstoppable, but we don't have to scatter ourselves in fragments along the way. When we include the whole internal community, we feel more whole.

Tips on Unblending

- Unblending is the whole ball game.
  - Pay attention to unblending above all. Once parts unblend, the client's Self can take over, and you can be an auxiliary helper, there to assist if a part blends and the client's Self isn't available.
    - Accordingly, your main job is to invite protective parts to unblend, and then listen, honor, validate, serve (by addressing their fears), and coax them into giving it a try.
- Age matters.
  - Ask parts how old they are, then gear your approach to what you know about that age group.
- The psyche contains a complex, multi-age community of parts who have suffered different losses and have different roles, perspectives,

experiences, interests, and gifts. Valuing some over others leads to conflict and a sense of fragmentation. Welcoming all of them invites good guidance and brings peace of mind.

Tips on Unblending Challenges

Protectors Speaking for and about Exiles

To forestall protectors from speaking for exiles, I say early on that therapy is a democracy. Each part is the expert on its own experience and can speak for itself. This rule asserts the equal value and importance of exiled parts and gets everyone's attention. I've never had any pushback, probably because the rule seems fair to protectors and applies to them as well. Of course, no pushback does not mean no interruptions. Inevitably, protectors continue to speak for and about exiles as therapy goes along, but, having established the principle, I can remind them.

Secrets and Fear

Protective parts who keep secrets are afraid of exiles who might reveal secrets. They may fear ending up in court either figuratively, with family members, or literally, with the legal system. When I hear these fears, I remind them that therapy is not a court of law. We're not looking for proof; we want to know each part's experience. Later on the client's Self and their parts can consider what, if anything, they might want to do about it.

Unwillingness for an Unknown Reason

We've talked about willingness at length, so I'll just reiterate here that willingness is an essential ingredient of therapeutic success. As I've described, I often think of IFS therapy as improv theatre. But regarding willingness, I also picture a racetrack that has two starting gates. The first gate is for protective parts, the second is for exiles, and they are in a relay race. Imagine if the first set of horses in a relay race were to walk out of their gate and mill about ambivalently, eyeing the second gate with suspicion, while the horses in the second gate pranced with excitement, eager to sprint. If therapy stalls between the two gates, it's because we have not addressed protector concerns sufficiently. That's our job. When obstacles arise, we can only get curious. Am I blended with a reactive part? Would certain internal discoveries threaten some of the client's external relationships? Is the client's dominant manager loyal to someone other than the client? If all of the client's parts could speak freely, would the client suffer financially?

And so on. Protectors come to therapy navigating survival. I may challenge their tactics, but I have to respect their caution. They know the client better than I do. It's not my life or my risk.

Internal Systems Seek Balance

Managers and firefighters are always seeking balance. As with Sir Isaac Newton's famous third law of motion (*every action has an equal and opposite reaction*), inhibition and disinhibition are a package deal. We see this, for example, when the leaders of rigidly hierarchical religious communities pick fights with authority figures, as occurred frequently during the COVID-19 pandemic. We see it when publicly puritanical, self-denying individuals engage in some secret disinhibition, such as celibate Catholic priests molesting and raping children; leading evangelicals engage in outré extramarital heterosexual activity or have alternate homosexual lives; anti-abortion politicians pressure their lovers to have abortions; outspokenly submissive women pursue power by disparaging the idea of powerful women; and so on. Faced with a demand for ironclad conformity, rebellious parts start wriggling. They don't see their rebellion as hypocrisy, they see it as a life-saving necessity. Clients who engage in compulsive practices ranging from mild to criminal with substances, food, gambling, pornography, sex, and so on are manifesting a similar brand of this culture-wide struggle to achieve balance and manage vulnerability. We are them; they are us.

Countertransference through the Lens of IFS

From the perspective of IFS, the internal system of parts operates by the same principles in you, me, and our clients. Countertransference may involve one of your protectors exiling another part internally and then rejecting a similar part of the client. Alternatively, one of your protectors might polarize with one of the client's protectors; one of your protectors might identify and side with one of the client's protectors; you might have a parentified part who feels responsible for the client; or you might find an exile who empathizes and identifies with one of the client's exiles. If therapy is stuck, check in with your own parts first (Redfern, 2022).

The Repetition Compulsion Is Nothing New, but We Can See It in a New Way

The repetition compulsion, so named by Freud, is arguably one of the stranger features of human behavior. The Greeks understood it, and the Oedipal myth contains a warning that is relevant for therapy today. In this myth, a prophet predicts that the newborn son of King Laius and Queen

Jocasta, Oedipus, will grow up to kill him and marry her. The king and queen respond by ordering a servant to kill their infant son. Instead, he gives the infant to a shepherd, who takes him to the King of Corinth, who adopts him. Growing up in complete ignorance of his origins, Oedipus does indeed kill his father in an altercation on the road and then marries his mother. Translated into parts language, this cautionary tale shows protective parts causing the future calamity they are trying to avoid. If you're skeptical about this assertion, think of critics shaming to keep an exile from feeling shameful. Of course, shaming reinforces the feeling of shamefulness and ensures a cascade of repetitive downstream effects. We can only avoid our own doom by inquiring (with kindness and compassion) inside and releasing (by healing our exiles) protectors who repeatedly tell us what to avoid and who not to be.

Talking about Parts in Psychotherapy Brings Big Benefits

As I've been saying, therapists who approach the psyche as a system with curiosity and compassion find many benefits. For one thing, parts are rarely hard to access. For another, as those who meditate will testify, it can be remarkably liberating to notice subjective experience without judgment. As clients chart the relational network of their inner system, the parts who arrived in therapy believing they were crazy—or that some other part was crazy—get a radically new and more inviting perspective on who they are. The client gets relief by hearing that rigid or acting-out protectors have legitimate motives and that exiles are stifled by identity burdens, but are valuable and good. Even if a person's exiles never unburden, this understanding can bring solace.

IFS Therapy Has Goals

Although clients aren't due anywhere else and they're not late for the future, IFS is goal-oriented. We aim to access our Self and the client's Self, forge connections with wary protectors, get exiled parts who are stuck in the past out of the past, and create the conditions (feeling understood, validated, loved, and accepted) that will cause protective parts to relinquish trauma bonds and inspire exiled parts to release shame-based identity burdens. The underlying assumption here, you have no doubt noticed, is that when the Self is consistently available, all this will happen as if the client has gotten onto a conveyor belt.

Strange Things Happen

Sometimes a client will come across what seems like an angry protector, but it denies being a part of the client's system and says it wants to destroy the client. Because an actor like this has an agenda for the client but is not part of the psyche, I call it an *outside entity*. I don't know what it is, but I take it at its word. If an outside entity shows up, the client may want to ask how it got into their psyche. It might cite an infected caretaker or some other relative. It might cite a time when the client was particularly vulnerable, emotionally or physically. Some won't answer this question, but the client has a sense of how it got in. In any case, hostile outside entities can't stay in the client's system if they're not wanted. Accordingly, we treat them like burdens.* Is anyone attached? If yes, we ask why and help that part. If no, the client's Self can usher the outside entity out of the system, giving it the option of going to the light. If this sounds like an exorcism, it does seem to be one. But as Robert Falconer (2023) points out in his in-depth exploration on the topic of outside entities and IFS, these evictions can be done with kindness and compassion.

Similarly, but with the opposite intent, some clients are visited by a benevolent nonpart, non-Self presence that offers wise advice. A benevolent presence like this might call itself a guide. If you're skeptical, as I was, I'll add that only a few of my clients have had this experience, all were surprised, and only one was cued up with prior spiritual beliefs. Whatever our personal beliefs, IFS is an experience-near therapy that works best when we validate the client's subjective experience.

Tips on Unblending Challenges

- **The Democracy Rule:** Protectors want to speak for and about exiles. They have an agenda and they want to control the narrative, which can be very inaccurate. Accordingly, I have a democracy rule (my only rule for therapy): Every part speaks for itself.

- **Secrets:** Protectors keep secrets; exiles reveal secrets. This big conflict of interest can stall therapy indefinitely, and taking a side will only make matters worse. Accordingly, we are careful to address protector concerns about what might happen if a secret were revealed before inviting exiles to reveal secrets.

- **Risk:** A protector may be unwilling to cooperate and also unwilling to say why. If that happens, our job is to be flexible and curious and to keep asking it to meet the client's Self. Protectors always have reasons, and only the client's Self can assess some threats accurately.

- **Systemic Balance:** You can count on inhibition and disinhibition being a package deal in yourself and others. If you only see one, the other is living its life in the shadows.

- **Therapist Parts:** In that we therapists have parts, and our protectors will have exiled our vulnerability in response to danger in the past,

---

*Hence IFS calls them *unattached burdens*.

we are the same as our clients. We know countertransference can be a potent obstacle in therapy; therefore, if therapy is stuck, we check with our parts first, and we keep on track by getting supervision and/ or therapy.

- **The Repetition Compulsion:** You can count on protectors recreating or reinforcing the calamity they aim to avoid (a.k.a. *the repetition compulsion*). The Self is a better bet.

- **Language:** Systems thinking—in our case, thinking in terms of psychic parts—is an invaluable approach to therapy because it challenges shaming, which aggregates (*all of me is weak, vulnerable, too much, too little . . .*), with parts language, which disaggregates (*a part of me got hurt and needs help*).

- **Therapy with a Goal:** IFS is goal-oriented. The aim is to access the Self (of client and therapist) and help protectors unblend so the Self can witness exiles, who can then let go of burdens and heal.

- **Outside Entities:** Some clients discover malign outside entities in their psyche. We don't do therapy with outside entities. If no part of the client is attached to it, the client's Self can send it out. But if any part of the client is attached, we find out why and help that part release its attachment.

- **Guides:** By the same token, benign entities can show up, giving wise advice to the client. Such an entity may sound like the client's Self but will say it is a guide. They're comforting and helpful to clients, and I also take them at face value.

Tips on Parts

Self-Like Parts Are Not the Self

Sometimes a client seems to be speaking from their Self, but the apparent presence of the Self is having no effect. Polarized protectors keep on quarreling, and exiled parts turn away. This signals that a manager part is standing in for the client's Self. We call this a *Self-like* part because it says the right things, sounds kind and compassionate (though perhaps controlling), and insists *I am Meredith!* (the client). A Self-like part will have learned to perform the role of the Self when the client needed protection, probably in childhood, and qualities of the child's Self were under attack. Self-like parts often worry that they will disappear or have no role to play if they make room for the Self. We can elicit this concern (*What are you afraid would happen if the Meredith-who's-not-a-part could help out?*) and address it (*You won't disappear, you'll just have more choices.*). Often Self-like parts need to be coaxed patiently for a while before they become willing to meet the client's Self.

Parts Can't Rescue Parts

Protectors fear being overwhelmed by the fear, shamefulness, and love-lorn longings of the parts they exile. When an exile feels crushingly alone and unlovable, protectors are afraid of being cognitively incapacitated and swept away by the urge to die when a suicide part offers relief. Because protectors are not equipped to help the parts they fear, we're not asking them for help. Rather, we ask them to stop doing what they do while offering to meet their needs.

Thinking Parts Really Like to Think

When a thinking part insists on, as it says, *understanding* why something happened, it is dancing around an answer that's already been given (and believed) internally (*it's your fault*), and it is preventing the exile from speaking for itself. Don't be led by thinking parts into focusing on content. Stick with process (*why do you do this?* not *what happened?*) until you have permission to help exiles. Focus on the thinking part's willingness to unblend and meet the client's Self. Keep guiding the client to do a U-turn so they can hear from other parts as well.

Dissociative Parts Require Special Patience

For many clients, dissociation is a defining feature of the aftermath of interpersonal transgressions or natural disasters. Nonetheless, anyone can develop a habit of dissociating. Just as some people are more hypnotizable than others, some have a greater ability to dissociate. Clients describe dissociative parts as, for example, clouds, fog, mental blankness, swirling colors, a blanket over the head and body, and so on. That is, they tend to show up looking like what they do rather than being personified. Bear in mind that the part may be a preverbal infant or a barely verbal toddler who will be challenging to befriend because its mentality most resembles a feral kitten.

Like most (probably all) therapists, I see a lot of clients with dissociative protectors who are very capable of and used to controlling the client's awareness. If a dissociative part won't talk with the client, it might talk with the therapist directly. If not, I assume it's preverbal. But if it will talk with me, I ask it to make room for the client's Self. If that doesn't work, I ask if any other part is willing to translate for it (a strategy I learned from Richard Schwartz) and hope for a volunteer. Sometimes dissociative parts work with (or for) other protectors. If your parts get frustrated when facing a wall of fog (as mine sometimes do), that's for you to explore. Remember, everything that happens in therapy is therapy. Every sensation, feeling, thought, or behavior in either you or your client is a player, and every interaction be a wrecking ball or a building block.

Critics Want Friends

When you're nice to critics, you'll be rewarded. Inner critics can be annoyingly persistent, and you can find plenty of advice about how to silence or defeat them in the field of mental health today, but they are actually well-intentioned and they desperately need help so they can let go of feeling responsible. Challenge their expectations by turning the table and offering to help them. Be kind, be curious, and ask them what they need.

The Word *Habit* Means *I'm Not Ready*

The concept of conditioning teaches us to view habitual behavior as entrenched and change as a slog. Protectors routinely promote the idea that habit prevents them from trying new things. When we suggest trying something new, they cite habit, as if we are asking the client to scale a glass wall. If we endorse this view, we're agreeing that an unmotivated, nonpersonified phenomenon, a mechanical repetition of behavior for which no one is responsible—habit—has taken charge and there is nothing to be done. If no one is responsible, there is no one to talk with about fears and needs. If there is no motive, we can't problem-solve. We're stuck. But this impasse is optional. IFS practitioners have plenty of experience with protective parts who've stopped doing something (even on a dime) when they no longer found it useful. We also have plenty of experience with parts who try new behaviors that promise to be useful, especially if they don't come with big risks. So, don't let cautious protectors convince you that habit trumps intention. It doesn't.

Firefighter Parts Pinch-Hit for Each Other

If treatment contains a firefighter part without addressing underlying, exiled needs and beliefs, another firefighter will pinch-hit. As one client said to me, *When I was in rehab for drinking, my eating disorder kicked up, but when I got to the eating disorder clinic, I started drinking again.* For this reason, we don't aim to stop problematic behavior; we pull out the linchpin by addressing its underlying cause.

Suicide Parts Soothe as Well as Kill

Suicide parts don't start off as determined, implacable executioners. Paradoxically, the promise that this pain can be stopped helps people who are in perpetual pain to function and stay calm. The caveat is that suicide thoughts, threats, and plans increase the chance of impulsive action in stressful moments. They also terrify exiles, who want to be loved for who they are, not executed for having negative feelings. Direct access is handy at any roadblock, but essential when a suicide part won't unblend.

Suicide Parts Scare Managers

Parts who threaten or attempt suicide govern our views of risk and dictate the rigid, fearful stance of people in managerial roles within mental health institutions (hospitals; clinics; treatment programs for addiction to substances, eating disorders, or gambling; halfway houses; insurance companies; prisons). It takes education, practice, and supervision for therapists to help their clients walk the tightrope between inhibition and disinhibition. Diagnoses that are associated with suicidality, especially borderline personality disorder (BPD), evoke a lot of managerial energy in treatment systems. The BPD diagnosis, which is mainly given to women with trauma histories, is defined very broadly in the *Diagnostic and Statistical Manual of Mental Disorders* (American Psychiatric Association, 2022) but features a core interpersonal dynamic of *come here–go away*. When I was an assistant director for a dialectical behavior therapy (DBT) program (a treatment for BPD) at a large community mental health psychiatry department, I saw many women who had graduated from competitive colleges and had professional jobs but were struggling to function.

In parts language, their young *I can handle this* managers, who were remarkably capable but had no practice asking for or receiving help, had finally collapsed under the effects of one too many betrayals, disappointments, or overwhelming challenges. Rather than evoking self-compassion, this systemic failure caused their inner critics to work harder and, as a result, they had little or no self-compassion. Their interpersonal injuries had taken root as identity and now, with more apparent failure, had grown into monstrously negative self-judgments. Meanwhile, their injured parts (exiles) were increasingly desperate. They idealized potential rescuers (*come here*), which caused their firefighter parts (who feared more injury) to intervene (*go away*). Reactive protectors (firefighters) tend to be more challenging for therapists. IFS is an appropriate option for high-risk clients with the BPD diagnosis (Schwartz, 2013; Sweezy, 2011), and it is also an effective treatment for complex PTSD (Hodgdon, Anderson, Southwell, Hrubec, & Schwartz, 2021), but what's hard in therapy is what's hard for you (Herbine-Blank & Sweezy, 2021). Be realistic about what you can handle and get supervision (Redfern, 2022).

It's Good to Feel Guilty
When You Should Feel Guilty

A guilt-based approach to relational injury asserts: *I'm not you, I've harmed you, I'm concerned about you, I care about being in relationship with you. I admit I behaved badly and I will take action as needed on your behalf.* This approach says two crucial things: *You are valuable*, and *I can do better.*

Forgiveness Opens to Many Trailheads

After a vulnerable individual is wounded, their protectors go to work with various tactics. They might criticize inside, be compliant in external relationships, or forget the whole thing; on the other hand, they might get angry, try to recruit others to the cause, or plot revenge. Unilateral forgiveness interrupts all this and signals a new plan. Rather than asking an external transgressor to take it back (because most won't) or asking them to heal the injuries they caused (because only the client can do that), we help the client make an internal offer their parts can hardly refuse: Let's get free of this. Finding and healing injured parts is the route to freedom.

Young Parts Are Literal

We've focused on shame and guilt in this book, and I don't think I'm exaggerating their influence on psychic distress. In fact, experience tells me that I've more often made the mistake of underestimating their influence. That said, a powerful event may be terrifying but not shaming. Whether it's shaming depends on the recipient's interpretation of the event: *What does this mean about me?* As this experience is different from what I've described so far, here is an illustration. In the following example, Aya describes a time when her grandmother died, her mother collapsed emotionally, and her father became enraged, which was scary for her at the age of 6. Her father's chronic rage was certainly shaming in other instances, but this experience, which is a reminder that young parts are literal, had an unexpectedly literal repercussion in her adult life.

● All Mothers Die

Aya was a 26-year-old, cisgender, heterosexual, Algerian Belgian American. She came to therapy because she was having panic attacks and dreams about dying. She had recently gotten pregnant by accident and was refusing to have an abortion despite intense pressure from her boyfriend, her sister, and her parents. She lived with her parents and did not expect to marry or move in with her boyfriend.

AYA: I had OCD and an eating disorder when I was a teenager, but I got over that. These panic attacks are new.

THERAPIST: Would anyone object if you talked with the part who panics?

AYA: Yes. They don't want me to get into that.

THERAPIST: We would ask the panic part not to take over so you can find out what's going on.

AYA: Oh. Okay.

THERAPIST: Do you want me to talk with it and you listen?

AYA: Yeah.

THERAPIST: Okay, I'll talk with the part who panics. Are you there?

AYA: (*After a pause.*) Yes.

THERAPIST: Would you like help?

AYA: Yes.

THERAPIST: Aya could help you. Would you like to meet her? (*Aya nods.*) Then you have to separate enough for her to show up. Okay? (*Aya nods.*) I'm going to talk with Aya again. Aya, the part agreed to stay separate and not overwhelm you. How do you feel toward it now?

AYA: I'm curious.

THERAPIST: What does it want you to know?

AYA: She's scared of dying.

THERAPIST: How old is she?

AYA: Six.

THERAPIST: Can you see her? (*Aya shakes her head.*) Do you understand why she's afraid of dying?

AYA: Meme, my grandmother who lived with us, died when I was 6, and my mother freaked out big time. She wouldn't get out of bed. My father has a big temper, and he got madder and madder. My sister and I lived on peanut butter sandwiches and played games in the closet with a flashlight for . . . I don't know. It seemed like days. (*Shrugs.*) That's how I remember it.

THERAPIST: What was the worst thing about that for you?

AYA: I remember Dad yelling at her, *All mothers die!*

THERAPIST: I see. And now you're going to be a mother. Is the 6-year-old confused about mothers dying?

AYA: Oh! (*A pause.*) I think that's it.

THERAPIST: What does she need to hear from you?

As this interchange illustrates, young kids are literal. It's always good to check with parts directly about their fears and ask how they came to have an extreme or strange belief. There's always a reason.

Tips on Parts

• **Self-Like Parts:** Sometimes a manager part is a very convincing stand-in for the client's Self. They seem to be cooperating, they may say all the right things (*I feel compassionate!*), yet other parts are unmoved.

That's because they know the difference between a part and the Self. The important point is that you may have to summon not only your confidence and patience but extra persistent diplomacy (*I know you've run the show and worked really hard, but there is still a John-who's-not-a-part*) to help a Self-like part unblend.

- **Parts Can't Rescue Parts:** Protectors fear the parts they exile because parts can't rescue parts. They can harass, smother, hide, and try to control each other, but rescue is a job for the Self. We're not asking protectors to *do* anything; we're asking them to stop doing.

- **Thinking Parts:** They like to think and they like to make up stories with neat explanations. We help thinking parts by (1) asserting the democracy rule (every part speaks for itself), (2) getting curious about process (why), not content (what), and (3) being persistent about asking the part if it's willing to meet the client's Self.

- **Dissociative Parts:** They tend to show up looking like what they do; they may be preverbal infants or barely verbal toddlers; they may work for another part; they respond to threats with hair-trigger speed; and they need kindness, patience, and persistence.

- **Critical Parts:** They mean well, are usually young (think grade school), can be annoyingly persistent, but are desperately in need of relief from responsibility. Offer them kindness and ask what they need.

- **The Word *Habit* Is a Sleight of Hand:** When a part cites habit as its reason for not trying something new, dig around for the real obstacle. Parts can give up habits in a nanosecond when they're ready.

- **Firefighter Parts Pinch-Hit for Each Other:** On the whole, reactive protectors work in a loose alliance, with one stepping in if another is forced to retreat. They are often trying to forestall death by suicide. For this reason, we view the firefighter part's behavior as a secondary problem, the result of years of trying to solve the primary problem ineffectively, and we offer to help with that primary problem.

- **Suicide Parts:** Suicide parts are comforting for other parts, as well as threatening. They offer hypothetical relief from the overwhelming emotional pain of being unlovable (and neglectable or exploitable), which can go on for years before an emergency comes up and the part takes action. When that day comes, however, exiled parts know they're up for execution because of their feelings.

- **Suicide Parts Scare the Manager Parts of Treaters:** Legal liability, self-blame, guilt, stigma, shamefulness, fear, failure, self-punishment, loss of confidence, and so on. You get the point. When we do not intervene successfully with suicide parts and a client dies, we face many possible persistent negative consequences, inside and out, personal and professional. Small wonder, then, that managers tend to take over when a client admits they have a suicide part. Unfortunately, inhibition spawns disinhibition; manager parts are proactive inhibitors, and suicide parts are reactive and can be uninhibited. Although we may need to hospitalize a client who is blended with a suicidal part, managerial energy raises the client's risk, and Self-energy lowers it. Our job with suicidal clients is, first and foremost, to stay in Self. Supervision helps.

- **Adaptive Guilt:** When deserved, guilt is essential to the project of being in relationship.
- **Unilateral Forgiveness:** When we forgive without conditions, we stir the pot inside and turn up important trailheads. It's a practice, not a one-time thought. If healing is your goal, try it.
- **Young Parts:** Like young children, young parts are literal and can misunderstand the present in ways that make an adult look mysteriously irrational.

Tips on Attending to the Body

Parts Who Shame the Body Have Trouble Living in It

A lengthy discussion about the body is beyond the mission of this book. IFS clinician/senior lead trainer Susan McConnell has written a book (2020) and a chapter (2013) on somatics and the body, and IFS clinician/lead trainer Nancy Sowell has written a chapter (2013) on chronic illness. She is also coauthoring a book on the same subject with me and Richard Schwartz. Jeanne Catanzaro has written two chapters on eating disorders (2017; Catanzaro, Doyne, & Thompson, 2018) and is writing a book on the spectrum of disrupted relationships with food and the body that result from cultural legacy burdens and trauma. For an in-depth discussion of the IFS approach to the body, I recommend their chapters and books.

But I will say a few words here. Shaming is a shock to the nervous system. Medical doctors call this stress, which we now know is intimately connected to physical illness, as well as psychic suffering (O'Rourke, 2022; Rediger, 2020). Shamefulness features in all the ways we disconnect from our bodies. Inner critics may attack the body for being too this or that, get angry with it when it doesn't perform right, gets ill, or doesn't fit their gender identity, punish it with lack of care or actual harm, or blame it for how it responded in moments of terror or sexual assault. People who were sexually abused as children may have parts who view the body as disgusting and dirty and who excoriate it for getting sexually aroused during abuse or, later on, during sexual encounters or at medical appointments.

The body is also fertile ground for protector polarities. Ideas about gender and biology spawn rigid role divisions and behavioral extremes. Cultural cliches about gender polarities have tremendous staying power. These include the polarities of compliant versus aggressive, emotional versus rational, dependent versus independent, prey versus predator, follower versus leader, nurturer versus disciplinarian, and so on. In the United States, rigid ideas about gender and sexual orientation that are tightly woven into the identities of individuals who follow Abrahamic religions cause followers to criticize and shame younger people who do not share their beliefs and who are asserting their own gender identities, sexual orientations, and sexual tastes.

In this way, American culture is tormented by its libertine-versus-Puritan polarity. As ever more graphic media depictions of nudity and sexual acts run back-to-back with incessant news stories about evangelical Christians working to rescind the sexual, marital, and medical rights of women, people who are dating and mating are enduringly confused. Adolescent girls and grown women talk to me from and about parts who consent to sexual acts without internal agreement. Men talk to me from and about parts who feel overly responsible or overly entitled in sexual encounters. Adolescent girls and boys down huge quantities of alcohol and cannabis to quell their awkwardness and fears about being touched or judged. Many people enter sexual encounters longing to be seen, feeling unseen, and barely able to tolerate being seen because their protectors fear humiliation, rejection, denigration, degradation—or being left out. Some dissociate from the body pretty much continually. Competitive managers compare jealously. Inner judges are brutal about appearances and pounds.

Yet the body is our home. It's our seat of emotion, the medium for relational intimacy, our vehicle for movement and action. Physical desire is enlivening, being desirable is sweet. Loving, feeling loved, admiring, and being the apple of someone's eye all bring satisfaction and contentment. Shaming is a huge obstacle to embodiment. Keep track of the body in therapy. You can explore how parts live in, relate to, and use the body, and you can interact with the body as an entity in itself.

Medicating Shaming and Shamefulness

Parts can use treatment for their own agendas. I've had clients who chose to get electroconvulsive therapy because a critic hoped it would silence wounded exiles permanently, and I've had clients who took anxiolytics or selective serotonin reuptake inhibitor antidepressants in order to quiet inner critics and soothe the parts who were being hammered by internal shaming. Medication can, of course, be useful. Some clients find they are better able to engage in therapy and life because of a medication that helps their parts unblend, whether the standard pharmacological fare or medicines such as ketamine, MDMA, and psilocybin. That said, the client's experience of—and need for—medication can change over the course of therapy. For this reason, clients benefit when we encourage them to track their medication experience. Frank Anderson (2013) developed an IFS-based approach for prescribing psychotropic medications, and John Livingstone and Joanne Gaffney (2017) developed an IFS-based approach for coaching medical patients as they make health care decisions. If you have clients who are navigating illness or taking medications, psychiatric or otherwise, I recommend their writings.

Tips on Attending to the Body

- **Parts and the Body:** This topic deserves a book—or several!—in itself. Luckily, some master IFS clinicians have written, or are currently writing, books on somatics, illness, shaming, and health from an IFS perspective (see the preceding citations). For the purposes of this book, keep in mind that a lot happens in the body. Exiled parts can try to show their experiences through bodily sensations; extreme protector polarities can play out in the body; and protective parts often try to use, change, or control the body to suit their antishaming and self-soothing agendas. Meanwhile, the body itself may be sending messages. All this calls for attention and the usual IFS manner of exploration.

- **Medicating Shaming and Shamefulness:** Protective parts can block the effectiveness of a medication if it interferes with their agenda (vigilance, depression, and so on), but they can also help guide a prescriber with information about the body and the willingness of other parts. For guidance on this topic, see the references cited previously.

Tips on Technique

Track Parts

If you take notes, you might want to devise a visually inviting way to follow the flow of a session and track parts. If you promise to return to a part, you want to be able to return. I have developed my own way of taking notes. I write the target part on left-hand side of the page, then I note reactive parts on the right margin. If a reactive part has to become the target part, I draw an arrow from it back to the left margin to indicate that this is now the new target part. Whatever method you devise, the main point is to have a way of remembering the part's story so you can return to it.

Language Is the Hammer and Saw of Your Tool Belt

As we've already talked at length about language being crucial in the practice of IFS, I won't belabor the point. But here are three reminders. First, you can talk about the Self without going into the philosophy of consciousness. Just say, *You have an internal resource that is not a part, and it can help your parts in all the ways they most need help. You can experience this resource by asking your parts to make some space inside.* This tells clients that the psyche is more expansive and resource-rich than its current crowded, conflict-ridden state would indicate. It also lets the client formulate their own ideas about the Self. Second, you'll get clarity on who is doing what to whom and why, by thinking of and speaking about parts. Third, win cooperation from protectors by using language that highlights the target part's agency. Rather than saying *She's blended with the exile*, try saying *The exile is blended with her*; and, rather than asking the client to *Unblend that part*, say *Ask that part to unblend*.

The U-Turn Will Take You to Important (Sometimes Unexpected) Places

If a client describes being shamed, ask this question: *When someone treats you badly, how do you treat yourself?* If we help the injured part first, then protectors calm down. If the client's Self doesn't intervene quickly, however, protectors will launch into a variety of strategies, possibly including trying to understand the shamer's motives, justifying the shamer's behavior, criticizing the exile, or getting angry and plotting revenge. While engaging in these kinds of strenuous, contradictory actions, the client abandons the exile once again.

Positive Reinforcement Is More Effective Than Punishment

Criticism and shaming are punishment, and punishment is shaming. Shaming is an aversive consequence (say, a public reprimand) aimed at stopping an unwanted behavior, but it leads to vengeful rebellion. In contrast, positive reinforcement, such as paying attention or offering food, aims to increase a desired behavior. Karen Pryor (2006) called positive reinforcement the good fairy of behaviorism. Internal critics use the bad fairy, punishment. In return, they get rebellion. Because they're tired and unhappy with this outcome (they really want social inclusion, safety, security, and happiness), they benefit from understanding how they can really be helpful. Although we cannot control each other, we can and do routinely influence each other. The good fairy of positive reinforcement—ignoring behaviors we wish to minimize while paying attention to behaviors we aim to maximize—takes discipline and the willingness to try something new, but it is the most effective way of exerting influence.

Welcome Skepticism and Distrust

I ask wary protectors to think of therapy as a laboratory experiment. They don't have to believe anything I say about internal resources, but they do have to meet the Self to find out if I'm telling the truth.

Unload Burdens as Soon as Possible

If your client is carrying a literal burden on their back, or in their arms, heart, teeth, joints, or muscles, they will literally lighten their load and get a sense of buoyancy when they unload that burden. After unburdening, the exile invites desired qualities to fill the space created by unburdening. But let's say an exile isn't ready to unburden at the end of a session. No problem. The part can opt to put its burden(s) in storage and invite those desired qualities in for a trial run. This strategy rewards partial efforts, brings at least temporary relief, calms protectors, makes it easier to return to the exile the next week, and facilitates the final unburdening.

Tips on Technique

- **Track Parts:** Take notes, or at least jot down some bullet points on parts at the end of sessions. Devise your own visually inviting way of following the flow of a session and tracking parts as you go so that you can return as promised. The point is to remember parts and the throughline of their stories.

- **Language Matters:** First, don't get hung up on definitions of the Self. Help the client experience their Self firsthand by helping parts unblend. They'll figure out what to make of the Self as they experience it. Second, be relentless about translating what clients say into parts language, which is optimistic, generous, nonpathologizing, and empowering. Third, use language that helps you steer away from implying that the client can control their parts (*get that part to unblend* vs. *ask that part if it's willing to unblend*), which may just rub a powerful protector the wrong way.

- **The U-Turn:** Ask clients: *When someone hurts you, how do you treat yourself?* and suggest helping the injured part first.

- **Positive Reinforcement:** Elicit ways in which punishment (criticism and shaming are punishment) have been counterproductive, and explain the benefits of positive reinforcement.

- **Welcome Skepticism and Distrust:** We want therapy to be a good, low-cost place for trying new things.

- **Burdens:** If an exile isn't ready to unburden by the end of a session, preserve enough time for it to put the burden in storage (if the part is willing). Then invite in desired qualities. This arrangement may not stick, but it's a good beginning.

Tips on Witnessing and Unburdening

Trying versus Doing

If a client says a protector is *trying* to relax or an exile is *trying* to let go of a burden, the part in question is not yet ready to relax or unburden. Either it's ready to do that or not. The protector who relaxes will get a better connection with the client's Self. The exile who unburdens will annul its attachment to imposed ideas about who it is. The part has to be ready. Unburdening is letting go, not trying to let go.

Exiled Needs

Exiled parts need to feel sanctioned, legitimate, and loved.

How Do I Know If a Protector or an Exile Is Telling This Story?

If a client tells a sad or horrifying story as if they're repeating a shopping list, I know that a manager who separates facts from feelings is hard at work and, at the moment, the client has no compassion to offer the exile. If a client tells a traumatic story and then stops to criticize or contradict themself, I guess that a protector is interrupting because the exile didn't have permission to speak. If the client tells a story that seems to have a lot of spin—for example, the other person is the only active character in the story—I'll guess it's a firefighter warding off a shaming manager inside, as well as potential shaming from outside. But if the client's story is rich in detail, like a good novel, and I feel moved by it, I'll assume the speaker is an exile. If I'm wrong, I'll soon find out. You learn to spot all this.

Transformation Happens

When exiles let go of weighty beliefs about their worth and heal their emotional wounds, the client may literally feel lighter. Often, their facial muscles relax, and they look younger, as if they're returning from a vacation rather than a harrowing trip to the past. I ask clients who have unburdened to observe and check on exiles. In trainings, Richard Schwartz recommends doing this for 3 weeks. The full impact of unburdening unfolds over time.

Backlash Happens, Too

The risk of backlash—the client suddenly becoming more symptomatic because their protectors activated to shame, frighten, intimidate, or in some other way punish them for making contact with an exile or for the exile unburdening—is higher if you bypass protectors at any point along the way to the exile. But even if you get permission to help an exile, the risk may go up briefly when the client's Self makes contact. Because clients who are doing well and feeling confident can feel blindsided by protector backlash at the last minute, it helps to predict this possibility and to keep checking with protectors as the client gains access to exiles. These precautions aren't universally necessary, but they don't hurt and they are important for some people.

Tips on Witnessing and Unburdening

- **Trying:** If a part is ready to do any number of things (meet the Self, relax back, stop overwhelming, unburden), it can do so. If it talks about trying, then it's not yet ready for action. Ask why.

- **Exiles:** Need to feel legitimate and loved.

- **Who Is Telling This Story?** Sometimes a protector will repeat a canned narrative devoid of emotion. This is a manager. Sometimes a client will tell a moving story that is rich in detail, like a good novel. This is the exile. Notice how other parts of the client respond, and notice your response.

- **Transformation:** When an exile unburdens, the client's physical appearance may change as notably as their mental state. Ask them to observe and check on the unburdened exile for about 3 weeks after the unburdening.

- **Backlash:** If protectors are concerned about exiles getting too close to consciousness, they take action. As backlash can happen any time, it's good to warn clients of the possibility and keep inviting protectors to speak up, voice objections, and participate in the process. Warn clients that backlash can happen and that it signals progress, not defeat. And get permission from protectors at every step of the way.

Conclusion

I hope this chapter will encourage readers to take certain things to heart in the practice of IFS. First, keep that all-important focus on accessing awareness in mind. It comes when parts separate so the Self can show up, and it is the golden key to healing. Second, translate your thinking and your clients' thinking into this conceptual model—that is, speak about parts—to get traction. Third, to automatically up your game in relationship with the client's parts, take them at face value rather than abstracting them into metaphors. For example, if your client has a question about a part and starts to speculate, guide them to ask the part directly. Parts are not an abstraction. They can answer if they want to. Along the same lines, try being open to strange information (such as outside entities and guides) and remember that the salient question about a client's experience is what it means to them, not you.

At the same time, parts who are afraid, young, stuck in a painful past, and focused inward have a limited, distorted perspective. Take what they say as information about their experience or agenda, not as a global truth about the client or other people. Their beliefs and behavior are valid for some situation—but often that situation was in the past. Although they are perfectly capable of unblending and cooperating if they want to, they are governed by lessons learned from bad experiences that have already happened and a desire to control the future. This is not a question of habit. We win their cooperation with respectful inquiry, concern, and compassionate advocacy.

SECTION III
Completion

Endings are an urgent concern in many therapies, and somehow or other therapy itself ends. Accordingly, we must consider how to end as carefully as we consider how to begin and how/when to intervene. Because of the discrete importance of ending well, this last chapter constitutes its own section. It is also my farewell to you.

CHAPTER 14

How Therapy Ends

There are many endings in therapy, and therapy ends differently for different people. In the United States, some people run out of insurance or money; some can only access time-limited therapy; some choose time-limited therapy; others have the resources to keep going in private therapy indefinitely. IFS has no set timeline, but there are useful ways of thinking about the time you spend with each client.

Stopping Too Soon

In IFS we always want clients to check with their parts before making decisions. If they decide to end therapy and we don't agree—we might think, for example, that their protectors want to avoid an exile—we speak about that concern and check on the client's willingness to reconsider. But we may not fully understand what's at stake internally, and, in any case, we don't have much leverage. Here is an example.

● Asia Ends Therapy

Asia was a 32-year-old, cisgender, third-generation Polish American lesbian who ran her own successful business. She came to therapy after ending a 5-year relationship that had become, for her, shockingly unhappy and conflictual. She described her mother as anxious, paranoid, and occasionally rageful and her father as distant, long-suffering, and passive. Toward the end of the pandemic, after 14 months of therapy, she said she needed to focus on her business, which was understaffed, and so she had decided to stop therapy. As it happened, she had also just made contact with a frightened little girl who hid under the table to avoid her mother.

THERAPIST: I got your message and I understand this will be our last session. I understand why, but I have a suggestion. Are you open to hearing it?

ASIA'S MANAGER: Yes.

THERAPIST: Two weeks ago, you found a little girl hiding under the kitchen table in your childhood home. She's scared of her mother and holds onto her father's shoelace. But she doesn't expect much from him, does she? (*Asia nods.*) Last week she began to show you some of her experiences. Do you remember? (*Asia nods.*) She showed you the time when her mother got angry and stuck a knife in the kitchen table. She showed you how happy she was to start school because it meant she wouldn't be home all day with her mother. And she told you that she signed up for after-school clubs and activities as soon as she was old enough because she dreaded going home.

ASIA'S MANAGER: I remember.

THERAPIST: She's scared.

ASIA'S MANAGER: Yes.

THERAPIST: She asked you for help. (*Asia nods.*) So here's my suggestion. Stick with her until she's ready to leave the past and unburden. Then take a break. If all your parts agree, it shouldn't take long.

ASIA'S MANAGER: (*Shakes her head.*) My business is in an emergency. I came today because it seemed right, but I just can't.

THERAPIST: Okay. Here's another suggestion. We'll put her in a place that's good for her, and she'll wait for you. Then we'll just check with other parts before we stop today.

ASIA: Okay.

THERAPIST: Where would she like to be?

ASIA: She loved summer camp. She'll go there.

THERAPIST: Let me know when she's all set. (*Asia nods.*) Good. Now, Asia, ask around. What do your other parts need before we stop?

ASIA: (*A long pause.*) They want to leave her at summer camp.

THERAPIST: What do you say? (*Asia shrugs.*) How about I talk with them and you listen. (*She nods.*) I want to talk with the parts who wonder why Asia shouldn't just leave this little girl at camp and forget her. Are you there? (*Asia nods.*) How many are there, Asia?

ASIA: Oh! A room full.

THERAPIST: What if Asia could help her?

ASIA'S PROTECTORS: What's the point of going over all that? We got out of there, and we won't go back.

THERAPIST: I don't want you to go back. But what if Asia could get the little girl out of there?

ASIA'S PROTECTORS: We want to forget her.

THERAPIST: Does it work?

ASIA'S PROTECTORS: Sometimes.

THERAPIST: But she comes back? (*Asia reluctantly nods.*) If she could be helped, you wouldn't have to worry about her anymore. Asia could help her.

ASIA: That would be nice, but they don't trust me.

THERAPIST: Okay. They need to know you better. I get that. Will they meet with you now?

ASIA: They'd rather leave. (*Glances at the clock.*) But I see the time's not up.

THERAPIST: No, it isn't. Will they give it a try? (*Asia nods.*) Ask for a volunteer. (*Asia nods.*) Ask the volunteer to look you in the eye and let you know who it sees.

ASIA: A vulnerable little kid.

THERAPIST: Ask the little kid to sit next to you, and then ask the volunteer to look again. Who does it see now?

ASIA: Nothing.

THERAPIST: It sees nothing? (*Asia nods.*) Ask the nothing part to separate from you, too. (*After a pause, Asia nods.*) Who does the volunteer see now?

ASIA: Me.

THERAPIST: How does it respond to you?

ASIA: It turned back to the others and pointed at me. They're talking.

THERAPIST: We can wait.

ASIA: (*Another long pause.*) They ask what I want.

THERAPIST: What do you say?

ASIA: I don't want anything.

THERAPIST: What do you offer?

ASIA: I can come back when I have more time.

THERAPIST: How do they respond?

ASIA: They'll think about it.

THERAPIST: Well, now we really are just about out of time, so let me say a word before we stop. These parts have seen you, but they need more time to get to know you. Meanwhile, they want to go back to ignoring this girl. They can do that. They can't help her, only you can do that. She's waiting for you at the summer camp. Remember her.

ASIA: Okay.

My biggest concern about Asia ending therapy at this point was for this exile, as my last words indicate. Because I didn't want her to be abandoned again. I advocated for her. It's more effective to suggest doing something than not doing something, so I stated my concern in positive, imperative language and hoped for the best.

Goings and Comings with Exiles

Whereas some clients end too soon, others finish definitively, and yet others complete a chapter of therapy and return later for another chapter. Some of these people return for a deep dive, others only want a few sessions, sometimes just as needed or every other week for a while. Here is an example.

● Raff Is Back

Raff (short for Rafferty, pronounced "Ray-ff") was a 62-year-old cisgender, married, heterosexual father of two grown daughters. He grew up in a large Irish Catholic family, with four older brothers and two younger sisters. His father was a charming, bitingly sarcastic man who was violent with Raff's mother on weekends when he binge-drank. When Raff was 15, his mother had a heart attack during a beating and died. His father sobered up and committed suicide 2 years later. Raff came to me to address a pornography addiction and fear of flying. He got to know his protectors and formed a good relationship with his exile. This young boy felt oppressed on many fronts and wanted to be the master of his own decisions.

A bunch of older-brother parts were pressuring him to unburden, but he refused, declaring that he wouldn't be rushed. Raff, who had lost interest in pornography and could get on airplanes again, felt confident that he could help the young boy and stay present with the older boys as well. I agreed, and he discontinued weekly therapy. If something challenging came up, he would call for a session. One day he called because he was afraid about having to get on an airplane to go to a big family reunion on the other side of the country. His head, he said, was filled with a buzzing panic.

RAFF: Why is this is happening again?

THERAPIST: Do you get an answer? (*Raff shakes his head.*) Where do you notice it?

RAFF: It's a high-wire hum in my head and like a big electrical storm all over my body, especially at night. I took a sleeping pill last night, which I never do anymore.

THERAPIST: How do you feel toward it?

RAFF: Well . . . terrified!

THERAPIST: Will it give you some space?

RAFF: I've tried.

THERAPIST: I'll talk to it, yeah? (*Raff nods.*) I want to talk to the electrical storm. Are you there?

RAFF: He's scared.

THERAPIST: Why is he scared now?

RAFF: Something to do with my sister-in-law dying. She was just 58.

THERAPIST: She just died? (*Raff nods.*) This reunion makes him think about her dying? (*Raff shrugs.*) Or he thinks about dying himself? (*Raff nods.*) What about that worries him?

RAFF: He wants to see his parents again so he can ask them, *How could you do that to us?* But he's afraid of pitying them.

THERAPIST: What do you say?

RAFF: I understand.

THERAPIST: How close are you to him?

RAFF: A few feet.

THERAPIST: Can you go closer? (*Raff nods.*) How's that?

RAFF: He doesn't want to go to this reunion.

THERAPIST: How about you?

RAFF: Oh, yeah! I've been looking forward to it. I like to see my siblings and their kids.

THERAPIST: Let's say you do go and he feels bad. What does he want from you?

RAFF: To hold his hand and say you're not alone.

THERAPIST: How does that feel?

RAFF: Comforting.

THERAPIST: What else does he need?

RAFF: He likes to know he's not alone.

I've had a fair number of clients with young parts who were preoccupied with dying. Like Raff's boy, they felt alienated from distressed parents who had misbehaved, sometimes extremely, and felt profoundly alone even in the middle of family. Although Raff wanted to go to the family reunion, the boy in him did not. A death in the family caused his young exile to think about the possibility of seeing his parents again. One of the boy's parts was angry and wanted answers from his parents, another part pitied and protected his parents. Raff had been listening patiently to this exiled boy, his part, and the parts around him for a long time, and their conflicts were not going to be resolved in one session. Because the boy needed quick comfort, I steered him to connect with Raff's Self and imagine having that connection at the reunion. This proved helpful.

What's the Point of Life?

Exiles lurk on the back burner of consciousness, unacknowledged yet coloring our mood and influencing our behavior. Endings provide an opportunity for them to break into consciousness. Here is an example.

● Hazel's Grief

Hazel was a 49-year-old, cisgender, heterosexual, partnered, Scottish English American therapist. She started therapy because she was in training to learn IFS and wanted the IFS experience. Her adverse childhood experiences included some bullying experiences with peers and her parents divorcing when she was 9. Additionally, her mother was now in poor health and would soon die. This session occurred shortly before her mother's death.

HAZEL: My mother is 88 years old and her quality of life is poor. Her life is over, I know that. But it's hard.

THERAPIST: What do you notice?

HAZEL: I dread pulling a tissue out of a Kleenex box because it might be the last one, and the feel of the empty box will be unbearable. I dread finishing a roll of toilet paper, or getting to the bottom of a jar of peanut butter, or pouring the last bit of milk. I never realized how many things end every day.

THERAPIST: How do you feel toward the part who feels this dread?

[*A U-turn.*]

HAZEL: Overwhelmed.

THERAPIST: You could help if it's willing to give you some space.

HAZEL: I hear *What's the point?*

THERAPIST: Of?

HAZEL: (*Shrugs.*) Life?

THERAPIST: Have you heard that before?

HAZEL: I don't pay attention.

THERAPIST: Would this part like to have your attention?

HAZEL: I guess so.

THERAPIST: Is it okay to pay attention now? (*Hazel nods.*) Where do you find it?

HAZEL: (*After a pause.*) Up a canyon.

THERAPIST: How do you feel toward it?

HAZEL: Dread. There's a rope coming out of the canyon toward me with a tick crawling on it. The tick is a messenger, but it disgusts me. I don't want to hear the message.

THERAPIST: What is the message?

HAZEL: It's going to say *life is pointless.* I don't want to hear that. I haven't been depressed since I was a teenager.

THERAPIST: What if you could help the part who is up the canyon?

HAZEL: Well, that would be good.

THERAPIST: Does anyone object?

HAZEL: They think there's no point; I should go away.

THERAPIST: Who do they think you are?

HAZEL: Someone who can't help.

THERAPIST: Ask the part who can't help to stand next to you. (*Hazel nods.*) Do they see you now? (*Hazel nods.*) Do they object to you helping the part who's up the canyon?

HAZEL: No.

THERAPIST: What needs to happen?

HAZEL: I need to go up there.

THERAPIST: Okay, do that.

HAZEL: (*After a pause.*) It's 9-year-old girl with stringy hair and dirty clothes. I'm listening to her, and she's not saying *What's the point of life?* she's saying *What's the point of MY life?* (*A pause.*) I heard it wrong.

THERAPIST: What happened to her?

HAZEL: Something about the divorce. I was 9. She felt forgotten.

THERAPIST: How do you feel toward her, Hazel?

HAZEL: I care about her.

THERAPIST: What does she need from you?

HAZEL: She wants to come home with me.

THERAPIST: Is that okay?

HAZEL: Yes. But there's a beautiful river in the canyon. We'll swim first.

THERAPIST: If she's ready, she could give her burdens to the river.

HAZEL: Yes. She's washing off that feeling of being forgettable. (*After a pause, nods.*)

THERAPIST: How is she now?

HAZEL: Much better.

THERAPIST: What does she need going forward?

HAZEL: Confidence. Love.

THERAPIST: Yes. Invite them.

When she was banished, the 9-year-old felt her life was pointless. When she asked about the point of her life in banishment, Hazel's protectors heard her asking a global question (*What's the point of life?*) and thought she was suicidal. Years later, they were still hearing her wrong and misjudging her feelings. Hazel could only learn that the girl was lonely, rather than depressed or suicidal, by paying attention to her rather than her protectors.

Firefighters Deserve a Happy Ending, Too

To wrap things up in therapy, protectors who have transgressed, inside or out, need attention, too. The ones who hurt other parts are mostly shaming managers; the ones who hurt the body and other people are mostly reactive firefighters. When clients see through the eyes of the Self, parts who have done harm don't seem bad. But they do need to be relieved of their jobs (which happens by healing the exile), and the client's Self needs to repair the harms they've done. Manager parts who remain attached to the idea of punishment (*That part is bad! You can't let it off the hook!*) may not approve of the client taking a benevolent stance toward firefighter parts who've caused problems. But compassion doesn't get anyone off the hook. Accountability and reparations are in order even when harms are irreparable in the standard sense, but they require persistence and commitment. Here are two examples.

● Walter's Irreparable Harm

Walter, a 63-year-old cisgender German English American man who killed a young woman in a crosswalk while driving drunk as a teenager and soon after made a career in the Army, had avoided therapy and struggled with excessive drinking for decades. Twice divorced, he had two adult children who wouldn't speak to him. After he retired from the Army, his girlfriend urged him to try therapy, and Walter finally agreed.

WALTER: How do you make it right if it can't be right?

THERAPIST: What do you hear?

WALTER: It can't be done.

THERAPIST: And when you hear that, what happens?

WALTER: I want a drink.

THERAPIST: So, if I'm hearing right, when one part poses the question *What can I do to make a repair?*, another part says you can't, and another drinks, or at least wants a drink. (*Walter nods.*) And what do you hear between *You can't make it right* and *Let's have a drink?*

WALTER: *Shoot yourself.*

THERAPIST: Which of these parts needs attention first?

WALTER: I don't know.

THERAPIST: Let's invite them all to a summit meeting with you. Are they willing? (*Walter nods.*) Are you with them? (*Walter nods.*) Do they see you?

WALTER: No.

THERAPIST: Would they like to see you?

WALTER: No.

THERAPIST: Who do they think you are?

WALTER: A drunk.

THERAPIST: Ask the drunk part to sit in a chair next to you so they can see you. (*Walter nods.*) How do they respond?

WALTER: They don't know me.

THERAPIST: What do you say to them?

WALTER: Hey! I'm here. You guys haven't figured this out. Maybe I can help. Why blackball me?

THERAPIST: What do they say?

WALTER: They're interested.

THERAPIST: Ask who needs your attention first.

WALTER: The guy who says I can't do anything.

THERAPIST: How do you feel toward him?

WALTER: I don't like him.

THERAPIST: Would the part who doesn't like him let you talk with him? (*Walter nods.*) How do you feel now?

WALTER: I'm asking *What makes you so sure I can't help?*

THERAPIST: And?

WALTER: Should I tell you this? (*A pause.*) He yells at me *She's dead, you dumb fuck! Shoot yourself. You can apologize in heaven.*

THERAPIST: He thinks you're the teenage driver?

WALTER: I guess so.

THERAPIST: How do you feel toward him now, Walter?

WALTER: He thinks I ruined his life. And I agree.

[*Confirming that the angry part sees Walter as the drunk driver teenager.*]

THERAPIST: It's true you can't undo the decisions of an impulsive teenager or bring that young woman back to life. But let's do a thought experiment for a moment. What's a fitting repair for a permanent harm?

WALTER: I dunno. I wish I knew. (*A long pause.*) An eye for an eye, maybe. I mean doing something on the life side of the ledger. I was in the Army for 20 years, you know. Afghanistan. Iraq. But I never shot anyone. I'm certain of that. I knew I wouldn't hurt someone under any circumstance, but I didn't talk about it. They would have kicked me out of the Army.

THERAPIST: Let's keep going with this experiment. That decision was on the life side of the ledger. What are you going to do next?

WALTER: (*A few beats.*) Take care of animals?

THERAPIST: How does that sound?

WALTER: (*Tearful.*) Yeah. I'd be grateful. I love animals.

After this session, Walter found a shelter for injured wild animals where he could volunteer. He also joined a group that traveled around the globe to rescue animals who had been injured in oil spills. He didn't stop feeling guilty about the death he had caused, but he did build a community and stop drinking, and he did feel he was making a repair every day.

● Trevor's Temper

Trevor, a cisgender, gay, Irish Portuguese American was 6′ 4″ by the time he was 13 years old. When he came to therapy at 41, he had been a heroin addict, a house cleaner, a musician in a rock band, and a fisherman on a boat in Alaska. He described having been challenged to physical fights often as a teenager, and he met the teenage part who had decided to be safe by buffing up with weight lifting and becoming scary.

TREVOR: I spent last weekend in jail.

THERAPIST: What happened?

TREVOR: I went to a fundraiser with Rory, you know, for his job, and this thing happened. (*A pause.*) I punched a guy.

THERAPIST: How come?

TREVOR: We were standing in this group talking, and out of the blue this guy looks over at Rory and cracks a joke about fags. And Rory's mad at me.

THERAPIST: Who needs your attention first?

TREVOR: I have a part who wants to get high.

THERAPIST: What does that part want you to know?

TREVOR: Well, there's the part who wants to get high, and then there's a big thing going on between the teenager who punched the guy and this other part who's like my age. He's just shaking his head like, *Will it ever end?*

THERAPIST: And how does the teenager respond?

TREVOR: Glares.

THERAPIST: How do you feel toward him, Trevor?

TREVOR: I pity him. I like him.

THERAPIST: Ask those parts to back up a bit and let you help him. Are they willing? (*Trevor nods.*) How do you feel now?

TREVOR: I do want to help.

THERAPIST: Does he notice you? (*Trevor nods.*) How does he respond?

TREVOR: He says he doesn't need help.

THERAPIST: What do you say?

TREVOR: We both know that's not true.

THERAPIST: Who does he protect?

TREVOR: You know I was 5 when my parents split up. I told you that? We got in the car in Idaho and drove to Arizona. When we got to this house out in the desert, we all got out, and my mother said, *Your father lives here now. Say goodbye.* We all just stood there till my sister said, *Where do we live?* Turned out we were going to California to live with her mom's sister. Dad didn't speak so we just hugged him and drove off. I didn't see him again for 10 years.

THERAPIST: The teenager protects that boy?

TREVOR: Yeah. He's 5, he's 7, he's 10. He's the bewildered boy.

THERAPIST: If you helped the bewildered boy, would the teenager be able to take a new role?

TREVOR: I think so.

THERAPIST: What would he like to do?

TREVOR: He likes playing the guitar.

THERAPIST: Good with you? (*Trevor nods.*) He's protected the boy. Now what does he need from you?

TREVOR: The other parts don't like him.

THERAPIST: Does he understand why?

TREVOR: No. He says he saved me.

THERAPIST: How about a meeting where everyone can talk? (*Trevor nods.*) Who needs to go first?

TREVOR: It doesn't work. They don't want to listen to him, and he doesn't want to listen to them.

THERAPIST: But they'll be even if they all listen.

TREVOR: Okay. He'll go first. He says, *Without me, you'd be dead ten times over.*

THERAPIST: What was he doing for everyone?

TREVOR: Keeping me from getting crushed.

THERAPIST: Do they get that?

TREVOR: Yeah. They know how bad it was in high school. But they still think he's an overactive bully. They want him to calm down.

THERAPIST: Would he be open to hearing what you want for him? (*Trevor nods.*) What do you say?

TREVOR: I want him to be able to relax and play the guitar.

THERAPIST: How does that sound to him?

TREVOR: It would be great.

THERAPIST: Okay. Ask the other parts to look at him again. He's a teenager who wants to relax, play the guitar, and let someone else be responsible. He got stuck in a tough job, he was heroic, but he wants out. Do they want that for him? (*Trevor nods.*) If he lets you help the bewildered boy, are they willing to accept him?

TREVOR: If.

THERAPIST: Right. Everyone has to hold up their end of the deal. What does he say?

TREVOR: He says, *You, too.*

THERAPIST: He means you have to help the bewildered boy? (*Trevor nods.*) Absolutely. Is everyone willing to try something new if you help the bewildered boy?

TREVOR: Like what?

THERAPIST: What we're talking about. He'd trust you and wouldn't take over, and they'd stop criticizing him while you do whatever you have to do to handle this legal case.

TREVOR: Okay. They'll try.

Trevor was a bewildered boy who grew to be an outsized teenager in large public high school where he was often physically attacked by other boys. As a result, one of his protectors became proactively tough and violent. At the same time, he had strong managers who helped him get off heroin, keep a job, and be in a supportive relationship. His managers were responsible, hardworking, and sincere about being good partners. They didn't like the angry teenager and were exasperated about his willingness to get into fistfights. I also worried that he would hurt someone seriously and end up in prison. Although the negotiation between the violent teen and shaming managers was by no means over in one session, the teenager did calm down and cheer up as Trevor helped the bewildered boy.

A Summary of Don'ts and Dos in IFS Therapy

Don't (worry about):

- Changing: Focus on willingness.
- Knowing: Ask.
- Problem solving: Wait.
- Working: Be curious.
- Empathizing: Be compassionate.

Do:

- Pose hypotheticals to avoid arguing with anxious, naysayer protectors.
- Redirect projections with the U-turn.
- Argue that protectors should try unblending and meeting the self.
- Clarify why the Self can help injured parts:
  - The Self is not a part.
  - The part isn't bad; a bad thing happened to it.
  - The past may not end, but the injured part can leave the past.

The End

As I mentioned in the opening, the IFS therapist, who is the Self for the therapeutic system at the outset, cedes leadership to the client's Self as soon as possible. The Self picks up an inner thread of fear and follows it through a well-guarded maze toward an exile, who waits to take the client into the wilderness of their childhood. If the exile is stuck in a bad situation there, the Self intervenes. *What needs to happen now that needed to happen then?* With this invitation, the exile takes charge, asks for help (if it wants), asserts its needs, takes action, and feels successful. Together, the exile and the Self rewrite and complete the bad experience, which, in turn, allows the exile to release identity burdens. In turn, critics and firefighters calm down. We invite them to move on to a preferred activity. Generally, they choose anything from resting on the beach to playing to helping the client in a more positive way. For some clients, a single unburdening is sufficient; others find exiles lining up for help. Though each unburdening is an ending, it may not be the end of therapy.

In any case, letting go of burdens and protective roles brings relief and grief. It's over. We celebrate! It happened. We weep. Everyone gains and everyone loses at therapy's happy ending. Exiles lose their burdens, and protectors lose their jobs; connection and compassion allow exiles to release their burdens, grieve, and embrace their gifts. We cry at the happy ending. Sometimes grieving means thinking about what was missing in a relationship; sometimes it means remembering what was given. Some clients have had caretakers who gave nothing; many have experienced a mix of generosity and emotional theft. As the giver leaves, we retrieve their gifts. Equally, when we say goodbye to a taker, we have the opportunity to reexamine their demands and say no. We lose, we grieve, we revive. At the very end, clients lose their urgent need for the therapist, and therapists lose their clients. We value, we care, we let go. When my clients stop, I miss them and wonder how they're doing, but because therapy is, as intimate relationships go, uniquely asymmetrical, they may not be in touch again to let me know.

Conclusion

I want for my clients what I want for myself. When they end therapy, I want them to remember that the shaming started outside. I want them to understand that shame is not an emotional still life; it's either the motivated external act (shaming) of an individual who is trying to manage their own sense of shamefulness, the motivated internal act (shaming) of a protective part who means well, or it's an exile's state of being (shameful). I want them to be prepared for vulnerable parts to get scared if someone shames them again. When a critical manager revs up—which it will on occasion—I want them to listen with kindness, remember how the part got its job, and be curious about its current motives. I want them to comfort their vulnerable parts even before their shamers. I also want my clients to understand the difference between useful guilt—the kind that gives us courage to admit the purposeful or inadvertent harms we do to others—and the misplaced, futile guilt they might feel even when they do no wrong. I want them to remember that they can't please everyone and that some bad things will happen regardless of their best efforts.

People come to me with their undeserved suffering, tricky temperaments, glitching minds, irreparable transgressions, and uncooperative bodies. Along the way, they introduce me to their hell-bent shamers, self-saboteurs, armored aggressors, and forlorn, orphaned children. I want them to love those parts, let opportunity knock, be in relationship, and heal in relationship, inside and out. I want them to feel that the domain of who they are is vastly greater than what happens to them. And whatever they're doing—when they get up in the morning, walk down the street, think, study, work, go food shopping, make dinner, take a bath, cry, or stare at the wall—I want them to feel loved.

References

American Psychiatric Association. (2022). *Diagnostic and statistical manual of mental disorders* (5th ed., text rev.). Author.

Anderson, F. G. (2013). "Who's taking what?": Connecting neuroscience, psychopharmacology and internal family systems for trauma. In M. Sweezy & E. L. Ziskind (Eds.), *Internal family systems therapy: New dimensions* (pp. 107–126). Routledge.

Assagioli, R. (1993). *Psychosynthesis: A manual of principles and techniques.* HarperCollins.

Bloom, P. (2016). *Against empathy: The case for rational compassion.* HarperCollins.

Catanzaro, J. (2017). IFS and eating disorders: Healing the parts who hide in plain sight. In M. Sweezy & E. L. Ziskind (Eds.), *Innovations and elaborations in internal family systems therapy* (pp. 49–69). Routledge.

Catanzaro, J., Doyne, E., & Thompson, K. (2018). IFS (Internal Family Systems) and eating disorders: The healing power of self-energy. In A. Seubert & P. Virdi (Eds.), *Trauma-informed approaches to eating disorders* (pp. 209–220). Springer.

Costa, R. M. (2020). Undoing (defense mechanism). In V. Zeigler-Hill & T. K. Shackelford (Eds.), *Encyclopedia of personality and individual differences.* Springer Nature.

Cramer, P. (2006). *Protecting the self: Defense mechanisms in action.* Guilford Press.

Csikszentmihalyi, M. (2008). *Finding flow: The psychology of engagement with everyday life.* Basic Books.

Falconer, R. (2023). *The others within us: Internal Family Systems, porous mind, and spirit possession.* Great Mystery Press.

Government of Canada. (2015). *Canada's residential schools: The final report of the Truth and Reconciliation Commission of Canada.* McGill–Queen's University Press. https://publications.gc.ca/site/eng/9.807830/publication.html

Herbine-Blank, T., & Sweezy, M. (2021). *Internal family systems couple therapy skills manual: Healing relationships with intimacy from the inside out.* PESI.

Herman, J. L. (2015). *Trauma and recovery: The aftermath of violence, from domestic abuse to political terror.* Basic Books.

Hodgdon, H., Anderson, F. G., Southwell, E., Hrubec, W., & Schwartz, R. C. (2021). Internal family systems (IFS) therapy for posttraumatic stress disorder (PTSD) among survivors of multiple childhood trauma: A pilot effectiveness study. *Journal of Aggression, Maltreatment and Trauma, 31*(1), 22–43.

Johnson, L. C., & Schwartz, R. C. (2000). Internal family systems: Working with children and families. In C. E. Bailey (Ed.), *Children in therapy: Using the family as a resource* (pp. 73–111). Norton.

Jung, C. G. (1969). The archetypes and the collective unconscious. In G. Adler & R. F. C. Hull (Eds. & Trans.), *The collected works of C. G. Jung* (Vol. 9, Pt. 1). Princeton University Press.

Kagan, J. (2010). *The temperamental thread: How genes, culture, time and luck make us who we are.* Dana Foundation.

Kelly, L. (2015). *Shift into freedom: The science and practice of open-hearted awareness.* Sounds True.

Khoury, J., Pechtel, P., Andersen, C. M., Teicher, M., & Lyons-Ruth, K. (2019). Relations among maternal withdrawal in infancy, borderline features, suicidality/self-injury, and adult hippocampal volume: A 30-year longitudinal study. *Behavioural Brain Research, 374*, 112139.

Klimecki, O. M., Leiberg, S., Lamm, C., & Singer, T. (2013). Functional neural plasticity and associated changes in positive affect after compassion training. *Cerebral Cortex, 23*(7), 1552–1561.

Klimecki, O. M., Leiberg, S., Ricard, M., & Singer, T. (2014). Differential pattern of functional brain plasticity after compassion and empathy training. *Social Cognitive and Affective Neuroscience, 96*, 873–879.

Klimecki, O., Ricard, M., & Singer, T., (2013). Empathy versus compassion—lessons from 1st and 3rd person methods. In T. Singer & M. Bolz (Eds.), *Compassion: Bridging practice and science.* Max Planck Institute for Human Cognitive and Brain Sciences.

Klimecki, O., Singer, T. (2012). Empathic distress fatigue rather than compassion fatigue?: Integrating findings from empathy research in psychology and social neuroscience. In B. Oakley, A. Knafo, G. Madhavan, & D. S. Wilson (Eds.), *Pathological altruism* (pp. 368–383). Oxford University Press.

Krause, P. (2013). IFS with children and adolescents. In M. Sweezy & E. L. Ziskind (Eds.), *Internal family systems therapy: New dimensions* (pp. 35–54). Routledge.

Krause P., Rosenberg, L. G., & Sweezy, M. (2017). Getting unstuck. In M. Sweezy & E. L. Ziskind (Eds.), *Innovations and elaborations in internal family systems therapy* (pp. 10–28). Routledge.

Lewis, H. B. (1971). *Shame and guilt in neurosis.* International Universities Press.

Linehan, M. M. (1993). *Cognitive-behavioral treatment of borderline personality disorder.* Guilford Press.

Livingstone, J. B., & Gaffney, J. (2013). IFS and health coaching: A new model of behavior change and medical decision making. In M. Sweezy & E. L. Ziskind

(Eds.), *Internal family systems therapy: New dimensions* (pp. 143–158). Routledge.

Lyons-Ruth, K., & Brumariu, L. (2021). Emerging child competencies and personality pathology: Toward a developmental cascade model of BPD. *Current Opinion in Psychology, 37,* 32–38.

Maehle, G. (2006). *Ashtanga Yoga: Practice and philosophy.* New World Library.

McConnell, S. (2013). Embodying the internal family. In M. Sweezy & E. L. Ziskind (Eds.), *Internal family systems therapy: New dimensions* (pp. 90–106). Routledge.

McConnell, S. (2020). *Somatic internal family systems therapy: Awareness, breath, resonance, movement, and touch in practice.* North Atlantic Books.

Mindful Living Community. (2021). *The difference between empathy and compassion by Matthieu Ricard* [Video]. Youtube. https://www.youtube.com/watch?v=ebJTV5kTIU0

Mones, A. G. (2014). *Transforming troubled children, teens, and their families: An internal family systems model for healing.* Routledge.

Mustafa, N. (2020, December 15). *Why Rwanda is held up as a model for reconciliation, 26 years after genocide* [Radio broadcast]. CBC. https://www.cbc.ca/radio/ideas/why-rwanda-is-held-up-as-a-model-for-reconciliation-26-years-after-genocide-1.5842139

O'Rourke, M. (2022). *The invisible kingdom: Reimagining chronic illness.* Riverhead Books.

Perls, F., Hefferline, R. F., & Goodman, P. (1951). *Gestalt therapy.* Julian Press.

Pryor, K. (2006). *Don't shoot the dog: The new art of teaching and training.* RingPress Books.

Redfern, E. E. (2022). *Internal family systems therapy: Supervision and consultation.* Routledge.

Rediger, J. (2020). *Cured: Strengthen your immune system and heal your life.* Flatiron Books.

Rochat, P. (2003). Five levels of self-awareness as they unfold early in life. *Consciousness and Cognition, 12* (4) 717–731.

Roubein, R., & Shammas, B. (2022, July 24). A triumphant antiabortion movement begins to deal with its divisions. *Washington Post.* https://www.washingtonpost.com/politics/2022/07/24/antiabortion-movement-divisions

Schore, A. N. (1994). *Affect regulation and the origin of the self: The neurobiology of emotional development.* Erlbaum.

Schwartz, R. C. (2013, May/June). Depathologizing the borderline client: Learning to manage our fears. *Psychotherapy Networker.* www.psychotherapynetworker.org/magazine/mayjune-2013

Schwartz, R. C. (2017). Perpetrator parts. In M. Sweezy & E. L. Ziskind (Eds.), *Innovations and elaborations in internal family systems therapy* (pp. 109–122). Routledge.

Schwartz, R. C., & Falconer, R. R. (2017). *Many minds, one self.* Trailheads.

Schwartz, R. C., & Sweezy, M. (2020). *Internal family systems therapy* (2nd ed.). Guilford Press.

Singer, T., & Klimecki, O. M. (2014). Empathy and compassion. *Current Biology, 24*(18), R875–R878.

Sinko, A. L. (2017). Legacy burdens. In M. Sweezy & E. L. Ziskind (Eds.), *Innovations and elaborations in internal family systems therapy* (pp. 164–178). Routledge.

Sowell, N. (2013). The internal family system and adult health: Changing the course of chronic illness. In M. Sweezy & E. L. Ziskind (Eds.), *Internal family systems therapy: New dimensions* (pp. 127–142). Routledge.

Spiegel, L. (2017). *Internal family systems therapy with children.* Routledge.

Stone, H., & Stone, S. (1993). *Embracing your inner critic.* HarperCollins.

Sweezy, M. (2011). Treating trauma after dialectical behavioral therapy. *Journal of Psychotherapy Integration, 21*(1), 90–102.

Sweezy, M., & Ziskind, E. L. (Eds.). (2017). *Innovations and elaborations in internal family systems therapy.* Routledge.

Sykes, C. (2016). An IFS lens on addiction: Compassion for extreme parts. In M. Sweezy & E. L. Ziskind (Eds.), *Innovations and elaborations in internal family systems therapy* (pp. 29–48). Routledge.

Sykes, C., Sweezy, M., & Schwartz, R. C. (2023). *Treating addictive processes with internal family systems therapy: A compassionate and effective approach for helping people who soothe or distract with substances, food, gambling, pornography, and more.* PESI.

Tangney, J. P., & Dearing, R. L. (2002). *Shame and guilt.* Guilford Press.

Twombly, J. H. (2022). *Trauma and dissociation informed Internal Family Systems.* Self-published.

Vaillant, G. E. (1975). Sociopathy as a human process: A viewpoint. *Psychology, 32*(2), 178–183.

Vaillant, G. E. (1992). *Ego mechanisms of defense: A guide for clinicians and researchers.* American Psychiatric Press.

Vaillant, G. E. (1993). *The wisdom of the ego.* Harvard University Press.

Watkins, J. G., & Watkins, H. H. (1997). *Ego states: Theory and therapy.* Norton.

Weilanga, C. (2017). *Rwanda and South Africa: A long road from truth to reconciliation.* https://theconversation.com/rwanda-and-south-africa-a-long-road-from-truth-to-reconciliation-75628

Weiss, J. (1993). *How psychotherapy works: Process and technique.* Guilford Press.

Zahn-Waxler, C., Radke-Yarrow, M., Wagner, E., & Chapman, M. (1992). Development of concern for others. *Developmental Psychology, 28*(1), 126–136.

Index

    Systems therapy
Inherited burdens
    concept of, 22
    letting go of inherited burdens
        exercise, 108–109
    obstacles to letting go of, 106
Inner critics
    offering to help, 249
    shame after unburdening and, 207,
        208
    shaming and, 9–11, 17, 24, 58
    treatment examples, 62–64, 87–88
    See also Internal shaming
Insight, 35
Instrumental shaming, 59, 60. *See also*
    Internal shaming
Intentional shamers/shaming
    behaviors of, 17
    dangers of seeing as beneficial,
        61–62
    listening for in IFS therapy sessions,
        118–119
    shame cycle and shaming others, 58,
        60, 66–67
Internal Family Systems (IFS) therapy
    burdens, 22
    change in therapy and, 23–24
    common problems
        activities of daily living, 236–237
        anxiety, 217–221
        depression, 221–226
        endless grief, 232–234
        fear of death, 234–236
        forgiving, 231–232
        major mental illness, 226–227
        racism, 227–231
    compassion in, 79, 133
    concept of plural mind, 1–2, 24
    concept of Self, 2
    concepts of shame and guilt, 15–18
    dynamics of promoting acceptance
        or change, 38–39
    ending therapy
        breaking of exiles into
            consciousness, 270–272
        goals of, 278–279

    protectors and, 272–277
    returning for more therapy,
        268–270
    the Self and, 277–278
    stopping too soon, 265–268
    examples illustrating the range of
        possible client experiences,
        10–15
    goals of, 26, 27, 37, 245, 247
    guidelines for conducting sessions,
        132–133
    importance of working with child
        parts, 2–3
    language and. *See* Language
    overview and key concepts in, 7–10
    overview of treatment portions, 27,
        115
    relationship between Self and parts,
        26–27
    setting the stage
        assessing the client's sensory
            experience, 130–132
        clarifying the client's language,
            129–130
        honoring wary parts, 137–140
        listening for shaming,
            shamefulness, and guilt,
            117–122
        overview and summary, 141–142
        starting therapy exercise, 125
        talking about parts, 122–125
        using alternatives to the word
            change, 127–129
        using alternatives to the word
            work, 126–127
        watching for and intervening with
            polarities, 133–137
    shame cycle. *See* Shame cycle
    strategies for maintaining flow in,
        115
    summary of don'ts and dos in, 277
    therapy as a theater metaphor, 140,
        143
    tips to avoid pitfalls
        on attending to the body, 254–256
        overview and guidelines for,
            260–261

Protectors
  addressing in the first portions of
    IFS therapy, 115–117
  apophenia, 45–50
  burdens and, 22
  change in therapy and, 23–24
  concept of, 9, 10
  convincing to cooperate, 47–48
  defense mechanisms, 39–41
  disowned versus owned behaviors,
    41–45
  dissociative parts and, 248
  distinguishing from exiles, 179
  dynamics of promoting acceptance
    or change, 38–39
  empathy and, 73, 74, 75–78, 81. See
    also Empathy
  ending therapy and, 272–277, 278
  goals of IFS therapy and, 26, 27, 37,
    245, 247
  habitual behavior and, 249, 253
  how to identify if a protector is
    telling the story, 259, 260
  intervening in exile–protector
    relationships, 177–179
  polarization. See Polarities/
    Polarization
  protectors can't rescue parts, 248,
    253
  recreation of the problem that's
    feared, 189–192
  relationship with Self, 26–27
  responding to the nonacceptance
    tactics of, 50–51
  shame cycle and. See Shame cycle
  therapist self-check on, 115–117
  tips to forestall protectors speaking
    for exiles, 243, 246
  trauma bonding and. See Trauma
    bonding
  trying versus doing, 259, 260
  unblending and. See also Unblending
    accessing Self and, 27–37
    balky protectors, 170–171
    capacity to, 36
    exile–protector relationships,
      177–179

  protectors recreate the problem
    they fear, 189–192
  when protectors won't unblend,
    32–36
  See also Firefighters; Managers
Psyche
  loss and psychic development, 242
  relationship between Self and parts,
    26–27
  response to trauma, 1
  as a social system, 1
  See also Parts; Plural mind
Psychedelics, 236n, 237
Psychopathology, defense mechanisms
    and, 41
Psylocibin, 237
Punishment, 257, 258

Race, honoring wary parts in IFS
    therapy sessions and, 137–140
Racism
  dynamics of inner shaming and,
    227–231
  racist firefighter part, 189–190
  treatment example, 229–231
Rape, shame-based trauma bonding
    example, 84–89
Rationalizing, 44
Reactive firefighters. See Rescuers
Relational burdens, 22
Relationships
  adaptive guilt and, 250, 254
  empathy and the parent–child
    relationship, 74–75
  intervening in exile–protector
    relationships, 177–179
  levels of protection in the Self-to-
    part relationship, 207–208
  of parts with Self, 26–27
Repetition compulsion, 244–245, 247
Repressing, 44–45
Rescript the past, rehearse the future
    exercise, 210–212
Rescuers (reactive firefighters),
    shaming cycle and, 56, 58, 60,
    67–69
Role plays, 192–196